THE LANGUAGE
OF AUTISM

THE LANGUAGE OF AUTISM

Understanding and Reversing ALL Symptoms of Autism

Pierre Fontaine RSHom CCH

To Ganesh, my Teacher and companion.

While writing this book, I listened to Puccini's "Turandot" hundreds of times. In retrospect, I like to think, Turandot resonates with the theme of this book as it marks an end to a time of darkness with wide swaths of misunderstanding and on the other hand the advent of a time where the light of clear understanding of autism at least creates hope. I certainly affirm that increased clarity is what this book brings to anyone interested in individuals or an individual on the Autism Spectrum.

As always, I express my very deep gratitude to all the parents who consulted me for their child and trusted that we would find remedies to improve or reverse autism. From the very beginning, I have enthusiastically done this work as much for the parents as for the children. I could not be happier and nor more honored to have made this choice.

Table of Contents

Overview

Nearly thirty years ago I decided to study homeopathy. I enrolled in a wonderful four-year program in England and studied passionately… I am still studying passionately. I chose homeopathy for its profound structure, precisely delineated and clearly enunciated Universal principles. I see it as the most perfect medicine. The substances we use from plants, elements and animals are transformed into individual nano-technology signatures that seems, even today, far ahead of their time. When taken, in the human body, each substance's innate qualities as a sum total of their effects replicate "in similia" on the physical, emotional, and mental experience and therefore heal. Only **Resonance** heals. This is nothing short of a giant leap forward in the understanding of healing in medicine.

I was happy that with homeopathy as my quiver and its remedies as my arrows I could fulfill my dream of treating dis-ease correctly albeit unconventionally and at the same time coming to understand the diversity and magnificence of nature to heal. Little did I know that autism would cross my path early, that my affinity to it be so overwhelmingly present that it would place me in the unique position of being the only homeopath to exclusively treat autism full time for over two decades. I could not be more pleased.

The nature of autism created a situation whereby the way of consultation had to be re-invented. My second book, "One Heart, One Mind" presents a new and novel method of case taking, I call "surrogacy". It is specifically designed to achieve depth in the treatment of autism. Illustrated by cases "One Heart, One Mind" presents the professional consultation using Surrogacy to fulfill the complicated task of "bringing voice to a patient who cannot speak". It is not a do it yourself guide to the reversal of autism. It demonstrates the depth, diversity, logic, and accuracy of homeopathic remedies and the great complexity of autism. While the breakthroughs described in the book are crucial to reverse autism deeply the method lacked ease of use. Without falling in the ineffective trap of the popular idea of "clearing" vaccines professed by some, which prevents depth, I was uncomfortably caught between a method that could pick a life changing remedy or create only minor changes. While grateful for the positives, I had to adapt to what I was faced with in consultation, I needed a more systematic approach to restore function on a wider scale. Carried by laser focused determination to only reverse autism completely, a difficult and extremely complex task, I endeavored carefully palpating my way forward, certain of the path but far from certain of any solution. With time the puzzle put itself together.

Homeopathy focuses on the patient rather than the illness. I felt I needed to understand autism itself much more. I previously defined autism as "total chaos". That still holds true but even chaos has order and a logic. While it took some time, thankfully autism itself came far more into focus. The answers to my questions came, and the methodology described in this book gives more rational options to improve, often enormously, the lives of people on the spectrum.

- The focus of understanding autism allowed me to discern the "Autism Modus Operandi" (M.O.) of the patient. Homeopathy's unique, multifaceted, procedure of analysis led me to clearly comprehend autism as a stage 12 condition, that is amply described in this book. Stage 12 defines and makes perfectly understandable the actions and reactions of individuals (on the spectrum). In other words, I came to fully understand why individuals react the way they do when for example they hear the word "no", a symptom that is present in nearly 100% of all patients on the spectrum. The rationale of it led me to help parents with the concept of "Parenting from behind".

Understanding the M.O., reveals some of the "secrets" and anomalies of autism. But that alone does not explain the logic of all the symptoms of autism. Modus Operandi is one aspect, what is missing is a true definition of autism. A definition, in a very practical manner should explain why a child prefers to poop in his diaper than sit on the toilet, or why a child can eat only one food, or why a child is interested in the credits of a movie rather than the movie itself. All these weird, highly challenging symptoms can now be easily understood through the very practical, new, and fundamental definition of autism presented in this book. This is a major breakthrough I am very excited about.

One thing leading to another, I also expanded the understanding of reversing autism beyond restoring spontaneous eye contact, interaction, and speech. I used to, very colloquially, term this "The three-legged stool" of autism but I realized that these three areas can be manipulated with control of the individual. What I look for now is what I call "interstitial space" that comes straight out of the new definition presented here. That is what cannot be learned. One can learn a few words and manners, that is what Applied Behavioral Analysis (ABA) and speech therapy try to do. But words remain contextual, learned, unless they become conceptual. The same holds true with interaction and eye contact. Concept cannot be learned, when the child "gets" what is essentially instinctual then we can safely say that that child will not remain on the spectrum for long. With cases, this is what I wish to demonstrate in this book.

One advantage of being in practice that is so intimate with people's lives is that parents always present me with their grief. One consistent grief is "My kid's handwriting". For years, parents talked their despair to me about it, I looked at these pages from school and didn't see anything until… I did. And from the fundamental definition described in this book, the specific autism handwriting is now understandable.

Another advantage of being in practice consulting with people, is to be exposed to what people do for their children. Now, it is extremely rare that I hear of a novel approach to autism that fits the principles of true healing until I was introduced to functional speech therapy. It triggered an idea that developed into "sensorial speech" and now in addition to the homeopathic approach I teach parents "how to speak to their child on the spectrum".

I have always felt strong empathy for parents of individuals on the spectrum. From the very beginning, witnessing the daily struggles and frustrations was a major driver of my deep dive into autism. In the same vein as "sensorial speech", from the perspective of Stage 12; I started to share adapted parenting strategies. It became increasingly important and along with sensorial speech "parenting from behind" became a three-pointed strategy acting conjointly to reverse autism.

Eventually, these different vista points developed into "The Language of Autism". While delayed or absence of verbal speech is a symptom of autism it does not mean autism lacks language. Much to the contrary. There is language in absolutely everything an individual on the spectrum does, it simply needs to be understood. When we look at Egyptian hiero-glyphs, we don't even see a language. At best, we see beautiful carvings that trigger wonderment for what they represent and "how they were able to create so much of it 3500 years ago?" At worst we see one sided painting we denigrate into meaningless infantile representation. The fact is that hieroglyphs are a language that speaks in great details of Egyptian reli-gious beliefs, social constructs, and individuals. Autism symptomatology is not dissimilar to that. When a child seeks tight spaces, hides under a blanket it means something very concrete. When the child has a temper tantrum, he is saying something. When the child does not suckle, it speaks of something and the same goes for taking a bath for hours or watching credits at the end of a movie rather than watching the movie itself. All of what an individual on the spectrum does is meaningful, we just need to comprehend the meaning.

All symptoms stem from ONE source. What autism actually is. Once this is understood, rather than thinking of abnormalities we can more easily care and surpass the prejudice. Ultimately, with understanding, tolerance, appreciation, support, awareness, thoughtfulness, kindness, indulgence, and empathy we can more accurately treat. In many ways one could say that such an approach will move the mind to think in terms of a person with autism rather than an autistic person. This book gives many examples of reversals and unique moments that came with the application of these sensible methods and the judicial choice of homeopathic remedies. I am aware it is difficult to maintain this distinction in everyday life. Yet, it is important to remind ourselves of the difference to readjust our humanist equilibrium much like a mantra recenters our thoughts or a church bell reminds us of the time of day.

It is my hope, armed with the most accurate definition of autism, that everyone will understand autism far better than is currently recognized. I also hope this book goes beyond the approval of homeopathy and into the acceptance of medical policies for people who deeply need them.

"The Language of Autism" ends with the possibility of how to prevent autism. A multifaceted triage method composed of "red flags" that might, from before birth and thereafter, if the observations are accurate, lead to the prevention of autism. It seems to me, given the chapter on "The history of autism" that it was always present. Today, according to my observations, a stage I call "Prodromal autism" or "dormant autism" is there but due to certain events, the course of life is changed. I run the risk here of identifying in a Stockholm syndrome way to the population I serve but certain characteristics lead me to think, given my early life challenges; that if I were born today, I could end up on the spectrum.

Pierre Fontaine RSHom CCH
2023

CHAPTER 1

Guiding Principles of Recovery for Autism

My definition of recovery for individual on the autism spectrum is informed by the following results.

1. Return of spontaneous eye contact. (E.C.)
2. Return of spontaneous interaction with peers and adults. (S.I.)
3. Return of spontaneous conversational speech. (S.S.)

This is the goal I first set for myself. It is what spurs constant refinement of the consultation to arrive as often as possible to accurate remedies that will significantly remove those symptoms. I give these three characteristics the very colloquial name of "The Three-Legged Stool".

I am not merely looking for improvements in individuals on the spectrum. I often hear "We have been doing biomed with therapy for years and my child is so much better now". "That is good!" And then, I hear, "He still does not talk. Socially he is awkward, and school is complaining about his behaviors". That is simply not acceptable! I understand the optimism parents have, but I purposely remain dissatisfied until I hear far deeper improvement from them.

The search for accurate remedies is tied to the understanding of the autism experience itself. Albeit autism appears severely chaotic there is a logic to its symptomatology. In my humble opinion, it is not possible to just look at the symptoms from the outside and draw conclusions. Understanding autism from its innermost recesses leads to knowing why a 10-year-old child would rather poop in a diaper than go to the toilet. I fundamentally believe that without such a deep inner understanding all is to no avail. Full recovery cannot be possible because to reverse autism one must know what needs to be healed in the patient and not treat an idea or theory. Then understanding must be accompanied by methods of analysis to pick specific remedies. Understanding and analysis should lead to homeopathic remedies capable of releasing blockages to development and allow great strides forward in dissolving the autism bubble that causes so much pain, on the physical, emotional, and mental level.

The return of spontaneous eye contact (E.C.), interaction (S.I.) and speech (S.S) is what I call "Phase 1". However, I have been fortunate enough to receive children who after my treatment functioned very well for years with no or little limitation in terms of E.C., S.I., and S.S. but then as the kiddos became teenagers the parents came back to me due to lack of maturity. A case that comes to mind is that of a teen who did not know what to do with his belt. He didn't have to wear one, at face value it was simple enough to control, but the parents rightly perceived that the belt was not the heart of the problem but rather that it spoke about something deeper. It is comprehensible for a five-year-old to not understand the purpose of a belt but for a sixteen-year-old it is not, especially since he had been asked to wear it for years.

One might be inclined to think that such an issue is the realm of therapy and that all this young man needs is, to be taught where the belt goes once and for all. I beg to differ. Combined with other issues we can understand that the solution does not lie in teaching him what a belt is. There is simply no way of teaching all life situations to individuals who generally take things at face value to begin with. This is in contrast with some parents' optimistic statements earlier. It is not uncommon to find a child in a very supported and controlled environment to "do well" but still be a phase 1 kid. Once the individual is removed from the routine, the perceived chaos takes over and disastrous behaviors reappear quickly.

A case in point is that of a 17-year-old who came to New York on a school trip. The teen, who was somewhat "verbal" and "social", came with the class. His mom who accompanied him spent years framing his life so that symptoms would be under control. Unfortunately, the daily control gave her a false sense of reality which directed her to confidently enterprise that trip. As soon as they arrived in New York the boy panicked and pooped in his pants as he exited the plane. Catastrophic! And he pooped again after he cleaned up. He could not express himself at all and had a total meltdown in the airport. The family went back to California in a hurry.

Human development is an exceedingly intricate process, composed of millions upon millions of bits of information taken from our surroundings which, somehow connect seamlessly in our mind, through logic, maturity, observations, and experiences. We take this largely subconscious ability or process for granted. The first case with the belt teaches us that a Phase Two treatment is adequate in some cases where remnants of inability remain. It is no longer autism, but rather what can be considered the facilitation of human development. As such, a case is not dissimilar from other neuro-typical cases that always include emotional and mental components.

The "three-legged stool" is a valid measure and reference, but these teenagers' cases taught me to revisit the depth of healing. What kind of healing is happening? When a child improves from possible mindless spin-ning of wheels to joining others with toys, what has happened in between these points and where? The "where" is what I call "Interstitial Space". It is the space in which understanding happens. It is the space between turning the head when called and not turning the head. That space that does not make the head turn, that is physical, but it is complementary to the physical. Interstitial space might be called the mind, spirit, vital force. A five-year-old, improved greatly and very quickly after giving the homeopathic remedy Oniscus. The dad said, "She is starting to show that she wants to do her own things". "She seems to want to be independent" "She wants to take her own schoolbag. She wants to put her seatbelt on by herself. She is sleeping in her own bed. She also communicates what she wants with "Let me do it", "It's mine". She does not like us to interfere.

This is different from the way she was before. She just didn't care about anything before and never did anything for or by herself."

Of course, independence is a great development, but it is not the most important aspect of her improvement. This increase in development or rather ability also means that she has "far less tantrums" and "transitions are much easier". What is most important now is that her independence expresses itself in multiple and very different areas. This is what I look for to gauge improvement. The more I see this type of diversity in the depth of improvement, the more confident I am the child will recover. While I am happy with an improved "three-legged stool", I am far happier with the restauration of functions across many different areas.

THE WHOLE PATIENT MUST GET BETTER, NOT ONLY SINGLE BEHAVIORS OR PHYSICAL SYMPTOMS.

The idea of interstitial space is not an uncommon concept, the only difference is that I apply the concept to the general development of a human being. For example, I am a Frenchman who lives in America. There are qualities within me that will always be French. These qualities are ethereal, but they have very real implications and influences on how I behave, my sense of humor, the way I speak, or react and accept or not events around me. At the same time, I feel very close to Ganesh, the elephant headed Indian deity as stated on the first page of this book, but my relationship with Ganesh will never be the same as an East Indian who grows up seeing temples dedicated to him, observing the intensity and faith of people giving offerings, hearing prayers, and listening to conversation about him. There is an invisible space between all this that makes life experiential and therefore contributes to individual development. I recently saw an ad on the New York subway for a skin care company, "Peach and Lily", the slogan said, "My wrinkles are part of my experiences, and I value those experiences more than I value the idea of staying young forever". Those wrinkles are a precise mirror of the situations that created individual experiences. All facets of our lives are filled with this ethereal matter, filtered through our environment and senses that makes us understand our lives in unique ways.

In the case of autism, we are confronted with problems of very basic inability attributes that apply generically to all of us. We don't think of making eye contact we do it automatically. We socialize, interact, and automatically speak. In a very linear manner, therapies attempt to compensate for the lack of active interstitial matter. It not possible to learn all situations and trying to teach in this manner can only further exhaust and frustrate the child. Therefore, when I see children on the spectrum make far larger connections as in the example with the girl affirming her independence in many ways, it gives me much optimism that the child will continue to improve, lose the diagnosis and be able to function in the world without any problems.

CHAPTER 2

The History of Autism Prior to 1799, a Turning Point, to Today

I n all areas of life, to prevent repeating mistakes and know where we are going, it is useful to understand history. Compared to other illnesses, the history of autism is particularly fuzzy. The Diagnostic and Statistical Manual of Mental disorders, (DSM) definition of autism has consistently changed through each of its different editions since its inception in 1952.

Most commonly, autism is thought to have first been observed by Leo Kanner. In his famous 1943 article *"Autistic Disturbances of affective contact"* he describes eleven cases of autism, all of them not dissimilar in their symptomatology to the cases we see today. Dr Kanner described symptoms of echolalia and desires for keeping routines with difficult behaviors. He made a note that the children appeared to be above average in intelligence and that the parents were particularly highly educated. This seemed to lead Dr Kanner towards thinking that autism was an emotional disturbance rather than a developmental or cognitive delay. His research led the definition of autism in the DSM-II to be defined as "childhood schizophrenia" with "atypical and withdrawn behavior".

While Dr Kanner's article spurred the term 'autism" to be included in the DSM-II, it was Dr Eugen Bleuler, a Swiss psychiatrist who in 1911 first coined the term autism from the Greek "autos" meaning "self". Dr

Bleuler also coined the word "schizophrenia". From his observations, he defined autism as "childhood schizophrenia". A definition that was also promulgated by Dr Kanner, no doubt aware of Bleuler's work.

However, in 1926, Dr Grunya Efimovna Sukhareva from the USSR, two decades before Kanner's article as pointed out by Annio Posar in *"Tribute to Grunya Sukhareva, the woman who first described infantile autism"*, described six boys with symptoms fully compatible to ASD. Dr Sukhareva noted the sensory abnormalities in these children. A fact that was acknowledged decades later in the 2013 DSM-V. She initially used the term "schizoid psychopathy" but later replaced it with "autistic psychopathy", a clear step forward towards contextualization of the condition. Kanner, acknowledged her research in a 1949 paper titled *"Problems of nosology and psychodynamics of early infantile autism"*. Sukhareva's term "infantile autism" was only listed decades later in the DSM-III of 1980.

A year after Kanner's seminal article, in 1944, Hans Asperger, an Austrian pediatrician, described "autistic psychopathy" in four boys of high intelligence but with social interaction problems. Many years later his work and observations were recognized as different from "autism" and termed "Asperger's syndrome" in the DSM-IV.

We remember that Kanner made a particular and specific mention of the parents, father, and mother, being highly educated and "successful". As such he wrote that "the child's aloneness" was clear "from the beginning of life". In a subsequent article, in 1949 *"In a different key"* he gave his observations of the parents a more prominent role and began to blame "cold" mothering as being partly a cause of autism. In 1956 Kanner also suggested that "successfully autistic parent had a milder, latent form of autism which showed in full emergence in their children". With such erroneous theory, no doubt advanced out of frustration of not being able to connect cause, effect, definition, and effective treatment, it was only a short step for Bruno Betterlheim a controversial figure in the U.S., to take advantage of the situation and in 1966 term the expression "The refrigerator mom" which found great resonance in the public.

The DSM changed the definition once again in 1987 from "Infantile Autism" to "Autism Disorder". The current DSM-V updated in 2013 no longer separates diagnoses of Asperger's, PDD-NOS and others but rather includes all sub-categories of autism under the umbrella of Autism Spectrum Disorder (ASD).

1998, is a watershed year for parents of kids on the spectrum. The Lancet publishes a study that the Measles-Mumps-Rubella (MMR) vaccine causes autism. This opened the floodgates for parents seeking to find a reason or a culprit for autism. Thimerosal, a mercury-based preservative present in the vaccines was advanced as the cause for autism. Of course, the correlation did not fall in deaf ears that one the first reported cases by Dr Kanner was that of parents conducting research on antifungal agricultural products using mercury. The connection between mercury and autism seemed to be established. The Lancet, caught between a rock and a hard place took twelve years to fully retract the article.

Parents often blame vaccines as the cause of autism. Are they right or wrong? When a case is properly taken, starting during pregnancy, those assertions often diminish, one can see that there were undetected signs that something was amiss, but it still does not mean either side is wrong. It seems to me that vaccines can be an additional factor in some cases, what I call a pushover, but precursors of autism are generally already there. So strictly speaking, vaccines, in most cases don't cause autism. It is important to understand that autism is caused by an array of problems, interferences, and precursors.

In 2000, I watched congressional testimonies conducted by Senator Dan Burton from Indiana state "I watched my only grandson turn autistic after he was vaccinated". His prominent role in putting vaccine makers and FDA officials in the extremely uncomfortable position of defending thimerosal, one of the greatest poisons ever invented, in vaccines prompted them without delay to remove it from most vaccines. That did not stop nor change the rapid increase in autism. Both sides of this argument, continue to fight a deaf-ear battle that has devolved into mockery and insults. Neither side at this moment is offering valid options of research and investigation to conduct constructive studies. It certainly does not help anyone, certainly not future generations, to keep repeating falsehood, only because we believe in them.

It is often stated in the community that autism was first observed by Dr Kanner. In fact, Mr. Donald Tripett, obituary of June 15th, 2023, describes him as "'Case 1' in the history of autism diagnosis" (NYT) was definitely not the first autism case. Autism did not start with Dr Kanner's article in 1943 nor did it start in 1911 with Bleuler.

In 1799, over one hundred years prior to Bleuler's article, after many sightings, a boy of about eleven years of age was captured by three hunters in the Aveyron region of France.

From all we know about Victor, he was deep on the spectrum. Much like Dr Leo Kanner's patients, Victor presented with similar symptomatology such as rocking, seemingly getting "lost in his own world while squatting by a pond". He never learned to read, write, speak, or ask questions though a lot of therapies, kindness and money were lavished on him by the highest authorities in France. Much in the same way as today, hearing tests determined that he was not deaf. He made guttural sounds and pointed when he wanted something. "He liked to go to bed at 9PM, though there were no clock on the wall". "He takes a lamp, indicates the key to his bedroom; and gets very upset if we refuse to obey him". "He wakes in the middle of the night laughing and likes to rock himself". He ate only potatoes and nuts. Again, much like today's children happy with a single food and chips. I suspect he liked the crunch. All these symptoms and more were reported by Pierre Joseph Bonnaterre in *"Notice historique sur le sauvage de l'Aveyron, et sur quelques autres individus qu'on a trouvés dans les forêts"*, who took great care of him for six months before Victor was taken to Paris to be studied for five years by Dr Jean Marc Gaspard Itard. Most recently, Professor Uta Frith who researched this case, believes Victor displayed signs of autism. Serge Aroles, a French Surgeon who wrote *"The mystery of the wolf-children"* also believes Victor's behavior points to autism. All I read about Victor's comportment, behavior, habits, how he liked to spend his day, what he ate, what he was not able to do, what he was not able to learn, definitely reflect a child on the autism spectrum.

In his book, *"L'énigme des Enfants-Loups"* Dr Aroles, tracing back to 1304, not only points to the impossibility of an animal caring for a different species, but more importantly, he states that "the forest was the largest orphanage in the history of man". Victor was not the first "feral child". He actually was never associated to an animal of benevolence. Stories of children living in the wild abound but most of them are made up stories. Other cases were also mentioned by Pierre Joseph Bonnaterre in his *"notice"*. What matters here is not the belief that the children were raised by animals but rather the behaviors and abilities displayed by a handful of children on their own. A child found in Lithuania (with bears), another in Ireland (with sheeps) and yet another found in Hanover "seemed to have the same difficulty in speaking and learning how to speak just like Victor". Bonnaterre further described that "He defends himself by biting like the child found in Bamberg" and that "the child found in Lithuania also had difficulty eating a more varied diet than that of a very few foods". To me, finding a few autistic children surviving a short time against all odds in the wild after being abandoned makes sense. What we will never know from the history of man is how many children on the spectrum were "lost" in the unforgiving wilderness. What we can be certain of, is that once the framework of a medical system was established children on the spectrum appear, so this is not new to humanity.

The first thing to consider is that the onset of autism is not obvious to the parents. While it was not unusual for newborns with deformities to be drowned or left without food to die, a child born on the spectrum does not display physical deformities and if it breastfeeds, the baby survives the initial stage of life in the care of the family. It is entirely conceivable that after the first couple of years a "difficult" child displaying abnormal behavior would be locked up in a room never to be seen given the deeply religious overtones, simple beliefs, and prejudices of the time. Such child would have been considered a child of the devil, especially if the child were illegitimate. No doubt, the family would be severely ostracized and shunned as I saw myself in some countries just a handful of years ago. Though infanticide was illegal, the emotional, material, social and religious burden were so great that abandonment in the forest, most especially of children who behaved strangely was the least of all bad options.

Victor himself had many scars on his body caused by being in the wild but one scar across his throat and near the carotid left no doubt that around the age of three, he somehow escaped a murder attempt.

It is important to understand the precarious position of children and the adult view of them centuries ago. William Kremer of the BBC detailed the writing of "an assistant to the Venetian ambassador to England was struck by the strange attitude to parenting that he had encountered on his travels". "The English kept their children at home till the age of seven or nine at the utmost and put them out, males or females, to hard service in the houses of other people's regardless of how rich people are". Errant children taking care of babies in the street was normal. Far worst off, children from poor families were regularly send to clean hot chimneys. Kept naked, even in the cold, many of them died in their teens of scrotum cancers or respiratory disease from the soot eating up the flesh. I come from a region in France where "le petit ramoneur Savoyard", today, a cute little figurine of a child chimney sweeper but the reality was that according to Christian Pourre "From the age of five or six-year-old, children would crisscross France by foot with their master". The same holds true for castrati, mostly boys taken from poor Italian families, given the promise that their child would live a good life of theater albeit castrated to keep the high pitch voice and sing for the pope and kings.

Under such known conditions of abuse, was it so awful to abandon a child in the forest and probably die of a natural death?

Victor arrives at a particular time in history. He was never associated to an animal, he didn't eat meat, but only potatoes, either raw or cooked. He seemed to have never been far from a dwelling. He quickly becomes a sensation and was ordered by Napoleon Bonaparte to be brought to Paris. The interest in him stemmed from fervent, ongoing empiricist theories of knowledge in that reason makes us human and can improve our condition instead of beliefs from religion. The lightness of Baroque music is gradually replaced by the classical era. "I think, therefore I am" as Descartes stated. In the context of The Age of Enlightenment, the philosophers Jean Jacques Rousseau, Diderot, Descartes who reflected on such probing question: What makes us human? What distinguishes us from animal? The presence of Victor as a wild child was a living laboratory to answer these questions greatly influenced Dr Jean Marc Itard who took care of him for five years, in his quest to make Victor learn. A newspaper wrote. "The people of Paris believed he was a 'noble savage of higher consciousness', then once they saw him, they said the exact opposite" which is not so dissimilar to what we see today. How often do parents tell me they were successful in getting their child in a private school, only a few months later be told that their child does not fit the school and should seek education elsewhere. Itard failed in teaching Victor to speak but continued his work with the deaf and remains known today as the father of special education. A hundred years later in 1907, his research on pedagogic methods inspired mostly by J.J. Rousseau, in turn were the inspiration that galvanized Maria Montessori's teaching method of emphasizing independence and viewing children as naturally eager for knowledge given the right environment.

One can be appreciative of the interest brough upon Victor for all the research it unleashed and the influences enriching our lives even today; yet we can see that since then autism has continued to baffle generations. It has left great many thinkers at a loss and pushed many, I am certain out of sheer emotional frustrations, to make statements and conclusions far from the truth. We can see that very little has changed regarding treatment of autism. One very practical outcome of understanding autism from a historical point of view is that we can partially disregard some of the trendy, uninformed and erroneous therapies prevalent in the community today, that perpetuate thinking that is at the very least flawed. It is my conviction that until we collectively understand autism in its most fundamental way, not much improvement will occur. The DSM-V continues to change the "definition" because autism is fundamentally not understood. I believe the current definition is not one at all but rather a description, and that the one stated in the next chapter is accurate. Until then autism is truly understood, treatment of autism will continue to be a guessing game.

CHAPTER 3

What Autism Spectrum Disorder Is. A Definition

The DSM-V description

Ever since Leo Kanner published his paper in 1943 on 11 children displaying "a desire for being alone with obsessive determination on routine", there have been many official descriptions of autism to define it.

The last time the definition for autism was changed in the DSM-V, which outlines all mental disorders for diagnosis, was in 2013. That year, several conditions with features of autism but considered separate from autism until then, such as Asperger's, PDD-NOS, childhood disintegrative disorder (CDD), High Functioning Autism, were declassified to make way for the umbrella term, Autism Spectrum Disorder (ASD). To be sure, the practicality of these awkward diagnoses, PDD-NOS for example which stands for "Pervasive Developmental Disorder - Not Otherwise Specified" was to say in the least; dubious. A diagnosis with such an opaque definition that it didn't give any indication of individual's symptomatology became a waste basket term for doctors to avoid pronouncing the devastating "A" word to parents.

Here is the current definition of autism from the American Psychiatric Association: "Autism Spectrum Disorder is a complex developmental condition involving persistent difficulties with social communication, restricted interests, and repetitive behavior. While autism is considered a lifelong disorder, the degree of impairment in functioning because of these challenges varies between individuals with autism".

After the 2013 redefinition, "Aspies" as individuals diagnosed with Asperger's syndrome proudly call and consider themselves as "high functioning" became part of autism. The new definition ruffled feathers but to give a sense of "spectrum" and practicality the DSM-V again amended the definition through its 2022 text revision (DSM-V-TR) to include three levels. Surprisingly, while ASD was meant to level the field, the spectrum is now described with three "levels" which do little to clarify the gravity of the problem. Today, most parents whose child is diagnosed with autism rarely report the level. Paradoxically, each level has its own spectrum as well.

Level 1:

Requiring support.

Difficulty initiating social interactions, starting conversation, maintaining interest, and responding to others as would be expected.

Behavioral rigidity and inflexibility.

Organization and planning problems can prevent independence.

Level 2:

Requiring Substantial Support.

Using few words and missing communication cues such as facial expressions.

Social interactions are limited to narrow special interests. Atypical social behavior.

Noticeable distress when faced with change.

Frequent restricted and repetitive behaviors.

Level 3:

Requiring very substantial support.

Severe deficit in verbal and non-verbal social communication skills.

Repetitive behaviors like rocking or spinning.

Great distress and difficulty changing action or focus.

Interacts only for immediate need.

The NIH and the DSM-V official definition of autism tell us that:

"Autism Spectrum Disorder (ASD) is a neurological and developmental disorder that affects how people interact with others, communicate, learn, and behave. Although autism can be diagnosed at any age, it is described as a "developmental disorder" because symptoms generally appear in the first two years of life". (NIH)

According to the already mentioned, *Diagnostic and Statistical Manual of Mental Disorders (DSM-5)*, a guide created by the American Psychiatric Association that health care providers use to diagnose mental disorders, people with ASD often have:

- Difficulty with communication and interaction with other people
- Restricted interests and repetitive behaviors
- Symptoms that affect their ability to function in school, work, and other areas of life

"Autism is known as a "spectrum" disorder because there are wide variations in the type and severity of symptoms people experience". (NIH)

"People of all genders, races, ethnicities, and economic backgrounds can be diagnosed with ASD. Although ASD can be a lifelong disorder, treatments and services can improve a person's symptoms and daily functioning. The American Academy of Pediatrics recommends that all children receive screening for autism. Caregivers should talk to their child's health care provider about ASD screening or evaluation". (NIH)

A lot of information can be gleaned from these rather lengthy descriptions. Such as: An individual on the spectrum needs various means of support to assist verbal deficit, limited social interaction and distress when faced with changes.

These descriptions inform us very broadly of what an autistic person "looks" like or what can be expected from an individual on the spectrum. They do not explain specific symptoms, nor mention any of the odd symptoms at all. In fact, I have not seen any definition mention any of the one hundred common symptoms. What the NIH and DSM-V give us, are largely very broad descriptions rather than a definition. I think this stems from not understanding autism at all, they simply have not figured it out.

Some of the most common symptoms of autism are, at face value, so illogical that if one insists on looking at autism from the outside, without a doubt in my mind, it causes enormous frustrations in researchers, even banging one's head against a wall for sure which, not surprisingly happens to be a common symptom. Frustration causes people to find "refuge" in erroneous ideas such as "The refrigerator mom", "yeast" causes autism, "heavy metals" cause autism, and now we are at the ultimate retrenchment when we can't find a solution, "genetics" causes autism. While the genetic route is now pushed more and more as the cause of autism, paradoxically, highly structured, intensive behavioral, psychological, and educational interventions are recommended, in fact, we are not very far or perhaps have even digressed a little from what Dr Itard was doing 1799. Difficult indeed!

A New Definition:

This book means to contribute to settling a concise definition. In "One Heart, One Mind" I described autism as "chaos". That is still true and very much part of autism though it is not the central aspect of it as I thought, but rather the modus operandi (M.O.) of the condition. Chaos certainly is not a definition. The modus operandi is the coping mechanism of living with the symptom's autism causes. Chaos and its counterpart: control, are the action and reaction to daily situations and circumstances an individual on the spectrum experiences. All of us act and react to daily life challenges within certain patterns of behaviors so anchored within ourselves that we feel it is "who we are". Our M.O. is part of us in life and in illness there-fore, we act and react according to defined patterns. The chapter "Stages of M.O." speaks to that extensively. At this moment, suffice to say that autism M.O. is stage 12 of a continuum of 18 stages.

Autism is: **Conceptual Inability.** The official definition of autism as we have seen is "Developmental delay that affects how a person acts, com-municates, learns and interacts with others" which does not explain the symptomology of autism at all. Developmental delay is in fact, the result of conceptual inability. Developmental delay does not explain why a child laughs hysterically, looks at spinning wheels, wants to only eat one food every day of his life or tenses up his body all the time. In fact, it does not explain much at all. Autism is not a developmental delay condition; it is the inability that makes autism look like a delay. Once we understand even if only instinctively, Conceptual Inability, ALL symptoms of autism can be understood. The fact that it is not a delay is the reason cases can be reversed.

The source of conceptual ability is believed to be the human brain, particularly the prefrontal cortex, which is, according to allopathic medi-cine, responsible for many higher-order cognitive processes such as abstract reasoning, problem-solving, and decision-making. The ability to form and manipulate concepts is thought to be a fundamental aspect of human cognition, it enables us to organize and categorize information, make predictions, and understand complex systems. This seems to support my definition of autism since most studies shows autism as being mainly a frontal cortex dysfunction.

However, the precise mechanisms by which the brain generates, and processes concepts are not fully understood. There is ongoing research in the fields of cognitive neurosciences, psychology, and philosophy to better understand how the brain represents and manipulates abstract information. Some theories propose that concepts are formed through a combination of sensory input, social and cultural influences, and innate cognitive processes, while others suggest that they are built up through more basic cognitive mechanisms such as analogy, categorization, and abstraction. All of this is true. The only problem is that medicine does not have medications for any of it.

I use the term "material medicine" not to dismiss it but rather to be clear that it does not recognize a unifying force. From a scientific perspective, there is nothing "before" the brain and its biological processes underlying human cognition. The brain is the primary organ responsible for generating all concepts and processing information from that starting point in a controlled or not manner according to some executive function. It plays a central role in virtually all aspects of human experience, including reception, thought, emotion, and behavior.

However, from a homeopathic perspective, we argue that there is something "beyond the brain, a non-physical force, vital force some call consciousness. These are ideas that are not supported by sciences. What medicine has done is wipe the table clear of all thoughts pertaining to "anything before". Medicine is capable to answer what happens in the frontal lobe, but it does not answer the organizing mechanism in health or disease. It does not answer why the child is more interested in the film's credits rather than the film itself, a totally logical activity once we understand autism. As such, medicine can only deal with broad aspects of diseases rather than understand the personal aspects of it inclusive of its odd behaviors.

The homeopathic approach calls the organizing principal the "Vital Force" (V.F.) which creates the symptoms throughout the body. The vital force level is the level at which illness needs to be addressed through substances of similar action. The V.F. expresses itself in disease through individual, highly personalized physical and emotional symptoms. The homeopathic thinking of disease is, in the rather bizarre if not paradoxical situation of being more in line with genetic discoveries than medicine itself.

There is nothing in the world we take more for granted than concept(ual ability). Dr Myo Naing, PhD describes *"concepts are causal, primal, universal and constant while contexts are resultant, phenomenal, secondarial, and temporal"*. We never have to think much about it at all because from day one, we don't question that a baby breastfeeds, poops, sleeps, smiles and is going to learn how to speak. Eventually the baby grows into a toddler and his conceptual ability grows with him, smiles when he sees a parent and cries when he is hungry or fusses when he is not paid attention to according to the experiences his senses have constantly provided him even in utero. Then that child builds a house with Legos unknowingly relating them to bricks of a house because the Legos are conceptual pieces of building material. They become sheet metal of a truck if the intent is to build one. The intent itself is conceptual, the fact contextual. A couple of years later, she rides a bike and goes to her friend's house down the street. None of it is taught. It is innate, causal, and primal.

Everything that surrounds us fits within a universal concept that builds on top of another ad infinitum, little change can happen within this evolution that started about 2 billion years ago with eukaryotes that eventually gave us life. A virus remains a concept unless it meets certain environmental condition under which it becomes contextual for us. If someone eats enough cinchona tree bark, that person will develops symptoms similar to malaria, not surprisingly the cinchona is a tropical tree where malaria thrives. If one is given enough mercury, then salivation will become abundant among many other symptoms, each of these two substances creates a sphere of symptomatology that become contextual to us but conceptual to the universe.

An individual on the spectrum lacks to a greater or lesser degree conceptual ability. The more conceptual ability is absent the deeper on the spectrum "level 3" an individual is. We are all flabbergasted when she sees a drop of water on her shirt turn into an uncontrolled tantrum. This, as all symptoms, is now easily understandable. Without conceptual ability a drop of water on her shirt is: a permanent fact. As such, it will always be there because the concept of past, present, and future, and that it will dry is absent. The drop is perceived as a fact forever even when the stain from the drop is gone. This perception combined with stage 12 M.O of "I must control this at all costs" spins into the experience that this stain must disappear right now and for that I must throw a major tantrum. Eventually perhaps, through habits that will create bits of contexts, a little event like this will create less of an upheaval but something equally uncontrollable will replace the drop of water.

The child passes bowel on the floor in the closet. There is no concept of toilet or toileting. Toilet is a thing. It is not a thing that is convenient and helps keeping me and my surroundings clean. There is no concept of cleanliness or convenience. Without concept a lot of children on the spectrum cannot see themselves or their family contextually within the world. Me and you don't exist; He and she don't exist and often even "me" does not exist.

When the iPad runs out of battery the fact is that the iPad does not work. The concept of plugging it in and recharge the battery is inexistant. Only after an inordinate amount of time (years and for most cases never) will the child, through familiarity grasp the context and plug it in but concept will still not be there... without homeopathic treatment. As usual, stage 12 dictates that in such a situation the way to go about it is to get upset, to illicit a quick response from someone in the vicinity for a quick restoration of a working iPad.

Socialization, speech, writing are all concepts. Socialization for a kid on the spectrum cannot happen because there is only "me" and as mentioned, even the concept of "me" does not exist at times. "Do you want a cookie?" and the child repeats an approximation "You want cookie?"

In this example, the child repeats so there may be a little bit of concept though it may be only a meaningless repetition without the sense of "me", of "want" and "cookie". Everything needs to be assessed to have as an accurate idea of where inability is the most pronounced.

I present for purposes of understanding "Conceptual inability", what "level 3" children on the spectrum experience. I have found that approach the most uncompromising and allows easier comprehension of lesser affected "Level 1" and "Level 2" by simply sliding the scale of inability.

Lack of eye contact is logical. Once we recognize that conceptual ability is absent, it makes complete sense that interaction with others is impossible. "Others" from that point of view are objects. Precisely what many moms have told me. One mom, I remember said "When he looks at me, I feel I am nothing more than a vase." In a "state of being" lacking concept, eye contact is not needed. There is no reason to have eye contact, there is no concept of it and cannot be an experience. A vase does not have a contact with another vase. Pulling dad's shirt to get some juice? That is something, eye contact is not. Eventually with a little contextualization, the child might look for a brief moment in the dad's eyes to get a cup of juice because "the vase has" grabbed his head with both hands to force a contact of the eyes, but it is not an eye-to-eye connection.

These moving objects make noise. How annoying!!! The next chapter demonstrates how annoying that really is. Language is incomprehensible. Speaking is nearly the ultimate concept. Language has purpose and can be learned but again without concept there is no need even though it is always there, which incidentally is the reason why a child on the spectrum does not use toys appropriately. Learning to speak with conceptual inability is… nothing, not even an idea. There is no concept that the sounds people make mean anything because meaning something does not mean anything. The concept that a language is learned is not part of their ability.

This definition of autism explains all symptoms. We can understand why reading credits of a movie is better than the movie itself. When a child can read, she has some concept. She understands the fact that one letter plus another form a constant. Letters are facts, much easier to put two things together than read human faces with its unlimited, ever changing and often contradictory facial expressions. Any word made of letters, is always a constant. Within limited ability, it brings some comfort. Knowing how to read, as is often the case does not mean there is understanding of the material read. A movie is the same, entirely conceptual, it does not bring any enjoyment, it is nonsense, it is nothing. Watching traffic cameras on YouTube, that is much more fun. It is perfectly logical that "Thomas, The Train" is so popular with kids on the spectrum. The facial "emotions" of that cartoon are extremely limited. They are so basic; they can be accepted with very limited conceptual ability.

When a child on the spectrum "writes" it is often our perception that tells us the child has written the letter "A" for example, whereas it is essentially a construct we interpret as an "A". Given the way letters of autistic children consistently look, to the child, I think it is three sticks. It is not an "A" or a "B" etc. Conceptual inability is the reason why the handwriting remains very elementary through the years. With therapy some aspects of life can be taught, like the routine of brushing teeth and some aspects of life can be somewhat better but the handwriting stays at the level of conceptual inability. When a child improves wholesomely then handwriting improves as well.

I bring the handwriting up because over the years, parents have consistently complained about it in their children, and they have wanted me to see it. For many years, I looked at the pictures of handwriting they sent as if I were in front of Egyptian hieroglyphs without any idea of what to see. I am a strong believer that when parents repeatedly point in a direction, they are sensing something. There is no knowledge of what it is but there is something. The same is true with vaccines. There is some truth, just not the whole truth and often it is very misstated. Then one day, I saw "something". It was an "e", or it was supposed to be an "e". I realized that the child was not making an "e" contrary to what everyone thought. It was like an upside-down Nike swoosh with a very short straight dash downward to give it an "e" appearance. The "e" was not at all closed and the downward bar was straight not attached to the tail of the swoosh. I noticed other "letters" with this little, perfunctory dash added to a scribble to finish or complete the letter. This looked like it was a two-step process instead of the one motion backward and forward spin a written "e" is. It seemed as if the letter was broken down into two components which meant that the child was not getting the concept of the letters. It was truly an eye-opening moment.

Then I looked at capital letters, they too looked very disjointed. The capital "A" I felt was really "three sticks". The two vertical bars generally not meeting at the top and the transverse always in different position. Again, it seemed the letter was not one whole but rather divided into three bars which now, considering conceptual inability makes total sense. There are two other common features when it comes to handwriting of individuals on the spectrum: Great difficulty writing on a straight line and great struggle writing small letters. To be sure, I checked dozens of handwriting pictures I received and indeed, most kids who write have similar features, at times with slight differences of course but all seem to be what I call "autistic handwriting". As the conceptual inability improves so does handwriting but not quite in conjunction with the improvement in eye contact, spontaneous interaction, and spontaneous speech. At this moment I don't have any answers as why there is a gap, perhaps it is only a delay given that written language is the most sophisticated skill humankind has developed. No other animal species has developed writing as a mean of communication. It is the ultimate, the pinnacle of communication, it therefore makes sense that it is the last vestige of remnant autism to disappear in the orderly reversal process, we in homeopathy take into consideration. We call this process, Herring's Rule of Cure that pertains to the direction of healing. It states "The cure must proceed from center to circumference. From center to circumference is from above downward, from within outwards, from more important to less important organs, from the head to the hands and feet".

As you can see, indiscriminate elimination of symptoms, read chaotic, is not the homeopathic path. We are the result of 2 billion years of evolution there is nothing haphazard in what and who we are, there is nothing haphazard in what autism is either. There is total logic and order to it and plenty of communication in all of what they do.

An inability, it is not an impossibility. Inability suggests within this definition that ability is dormant. With proper understanding and treatment, the potential of being able to kindle and grow the conceptual ability is possible. The root of the word is "Posse" from Latin "possibilism" "That can be done" or "be able", that something can be done by available means. With autism, at face value nothing makes sense. Only once we understand autism as a conceptual inability can we understand its apparent conflicts, contradictory and often bizarre symptomology. Only when an accurate homeopathic remedy is given can ability be restored most systematically. There are what I call "accidental cases" of reversal using detoxifying agents, such as DMSA or even some medications. Reversal has happened not so much because of detoxifying or chelating heavy metal but rather because the given agents have a complete effect on the individual.

CHAPTER 4

The Autism Experience
"Situational Autism"

The purpose of emerging ourselves in the experience of being on the spectrum is to acquire the sensation and thereby understand the logic of why individuals on the spectrum do, what they do. From the description of conceptual inability presented here we can expand from the theoretical aspect of the definition to something much more life mimicking, what I call "situational autism". Once we experience the symptomatology of the patient, we understand autism from its own interior. This prevents us from passing judgment that is consistently prejudiced as well as remarkably inaccurate.

At this moment what we know of autism comes from two sources.

1. The patients diagnosed with autism who describe their experience.
2. From research looking at the patients and drawing conclusions.

There are drawbacks to both sources.

The first does not relay the deeper autism experience. Certainly, the parents of my patients would be very happy if their child could write a book and make YouTube videos as those lightly on the spectrum can do. Generally, these relate personal stories rather than the deeper meaningful understanding we need to have to appreciate a level 3 individual on the spectrum. I have found such testimonials, often from "Aspies" do not relate to the whole spectrum at all. Singular and limited, often self-serving as in "I feel fine being on the spectrum, it is me and nothing can be done. I don't see why anyone would want to get rid of my autism". OK! As I said, not deep enough! I even wonder whether some of these individuals who claim to be on the spectrum actually are. Certainly, this level of suffering is not anywhere close to the cases I see. Although this "level 1" seems to be commonly romanticized in the media, these declarations are harmful on two levels.

1. Their affirmations minimize the gravity of autism and consequently prevent aid for those who need great help.
2. As Kanner alluded in his 1956 article, *successfully autistic parent had a milder, latent form of autism which showed in full emergence in their children*".

We know illnesses, most commonly tend to be transferred to the next generation in a more potent manner. Activated through the family line, a mildly autistic individual is likely to have a more autistic child therefore anything that can be done to heal will help the next generation. Furthermore, given how extremely challenging and patience requiring it is to raise an autistic child I wonder how prepared a parent on the spectrum might be to embrace extreme challenges.

It is worth speaking at this moment to the long list of celebrities supposedly on the spectrum such as Einstein (of course), Bill Gates, Mozart, Jerry Seinfeld, Michelangelo, Steve jobs and coach Belichick etc. As I am aware, none of these people have passed on autism to their children. Spending a lot of time at work, thinking monomaniacally about a subject, and wearing a hoody does not make one autistic. Again, such bombastic list, grabbing some of the most recognized names in the world to fulfill an agenda, dismisses and invalidates individuals who suffer very deeply and require a great many resources.

The second source is seen from the outside looking in which generally implies a black and white simplified and elementary logic. For constipation use probiotics because food today is so bad. For hyperactivity use Ritalin. In the worst-case scenarios, detox or "clear" the body of vaccines and heavy metals with dozens of rounds of DMSA or other chelators. The question: "How can a one-year-old child to be so toxic as to severely impede the most basic human functions?" is simply not asked, autism is not about heavy metal poisoning. There are many children worldwide growing up on smoldering garbage dumps and don't have autism. Many studies attest to the devastating effects of such environment on the children's health, autism is not one of them.

I understand that a homeopath questioning certain alternative approaches seems paradoxical. I do cringe when I hear of "vaccine clears", "strep clears" or Lyme treatment for autism using homeopathic remedies. Such simplistic approaches appeal to desperate parents greatly, there is no way of minimizing that. The idea that something can "clear" a vaccine is music to the parents' ears, big time!!! but that is simply not true and will never be true. When it comes to heavy metal and mercury, again, knowing history is extremely important. A little over 100 years ago, when people visited a doctor, they were given mercury to eat... so much of it that the patient would be told to stop once excessive salivation, a symptom of mercury poisoning, happened. Yes, that is true, that is why "medicine" changed its name to the term "Modern Medicine" used today as a way of sweeping that history of mercury and bloodletting under the rug. Yet, with all that mercury, autism was not prevalent at the time.

From the vantage point of Coneeptual Inability, we can then lean in and experience it. If you wish to experience it, I suggest you read the rest of this chapter as a deep dive once, then sit comfortably and retrace the description. Let yourself go as much as you can into the situational depicted here. You can do this again and again to extend your access to aspects you didn't experience in your prior tries. You are the baby, then the toddler, and finally the teen in the room. I help you at times to remain in that state by pointing out kiddo's point of view. Here we go? Read on.

Being on the spectrum, is like being in a white room. The color white is not harsh, it is mostly pleasant on the eyes. The room is rectangular, roughly the size of an average ranch house without walls inside. At times, the room is black (If you feel black fits more your situation then stay with black). The height of the ceiling does not feel repressive at all, about 12-foot ceiling. There are no windows or doors. It is never dark, even when the room is black. There is no sense of day and night. There is a faint sense of time of day, rather than time as a concept. The light is consistent, not too bright nor too dark. The same goes for the temperature, consistent and pleasant. There is no thought or idea of leaving or entering this room, nothing else exists outside of this room.

In this room there is a group of people, ten to twelve men and women seated at a table. The room is large enough to easily accommodate everyone and leaves plenty of space for comfort. From time to time someone gets up and stands for a while. They are always together, and always talk, not all at once but the talking does not stop. The group is not loud, they enjoy themselves but remain somewhat subdued. They seem to never sleep.

In this room there is also a baby who has no association to the group. He is just there separate from the group. The group is focused on its seemingly endless conversation, aware of the baby but it does not demand anything at all, it is as if it is invisible. He sees the group but does not feel any affinity towards it, nor does it have any sense that the group could help, nurture, safeguard or feed him. There is no warmth felt from the group, there is no sense of reaching out to it. Baby does not have a purpose to make its presence known, all there is from this group is it's incessant speaking, 24 – 7 – 365. The constant sounds coming from the group are quite irritating and are one reason for staying away from it.

At the deepest level of affliction, "level 3" conceptual abilities to survive are not even there. A lot of children on the spectrum have significant feeding problems from birth. It is quite common that they refuse the breast or have problems suckling the breast. This seems to be an extension of feeding problems in utero, as low birth weight is a consistent marker for autism. Often, they take the bottle rather than the breast with formulas that taste sweeter than breast milk. Dozens of studies show some association between breastfeeding and ASD, but I doubt there is a linear correlation to it. What I find interesting is the preference for the bottle which fits the stoical aspect of a thing rather than a mom.

"Baby" is paid attention to, he is well taken care of, but baby does not need much at all. Perfect baby. In fact, baby seems to entertain himself quite well. There is always distance, even when handled tenderly there is distance, all this care is not particularly pleasant, it is too much. At best the feeling is "give me what I want" but that is not the adults in the room are seeing it. It is important to keep in mind that all that we do with babies and toddler, the high "aaaa", high "ooooo", up-close faces, and the exaggerated faces with big eyes, wide open mouths we make are exactly the opposite of what a child on the spectrum appreciates seeing. Remember from baby's point to view "Thomas, the train" with its basic "plastic" emotions is appealing.

Feeding and transitioning to regular food remains difficult, eventually eating one or two foods is satisfying enough. With limited ability, there is absolutely no need for diversity at all; being offered more is very annoying. As parents we want to feed the child, it is our duty. For the toddler or the child, it is non-sense. I like this! I only want to eat this. Get it?

Over time, the 24 – 7 – 365 droning noises from the group incessantly speaking has become extremely irritating, to the point of being repulsive. The only thing toddler can do is to stay away as far away as possible from them. This is like being with a group of people speaking a different language. The only exception is that as neuro typical we will try to understand, the other party will try to make itself understood too, and at least socially there is an exchange. But after a few days, you don't like the sound of the language and you don't find an affinity with the people. Very soon you will be sitting on a couch looking at your phone with no desire to share at all. In fact, it won't take much time for you to start being irritated and spend days by yourself. Imagine that, for your whole life, every day with lesser rather than greater ability to comprehend, that is the autistic experience.

Eventually, so much effort is invested to help toddler, that somehow, within his scrambled brain, he senses there is something wrong with him.

Toddler is sitting in a corner, on the floor, hands covering his ears. It is best to stay away and try to not hear, just block the noise as much as possible. After a few minutes of high concentration to hinder the sound, he removes his hands, it is intolerable, the mind has been trained over time to diminish the sound, but it is always there, relentlessly irritating the mind, itself unable to process anything at the speed that is needed, it is the turtle and hare situation in the mind. It is inescapable and making the mind feel like it is literally scrambled. Scrambled is painful in many ways and makes him do all kinds of things seemingly without logic. Aggression inevitably peaks.

From this perspective of limited interest for what is around, the floor is interesting. There are simple things there, clumps of dust, a piece of paper or fibers from the carpet are perfect to look at. Those things are simple. They happen to be there just like that. Toddler lays down next to a toy truck on the floor. Toy truck is a toy, the sense – concept - of what to do is not there, spinning wheels on the other hand, just great, simple, consistent, and wonderful.

As life goes on, the people who give food, bath, and help to teach things contextually, are wanting to make kiddo learn more. but learning handwriting, speech, and various cerebral tasks, while spinning wheels is the greatest thing is extremely difficult to bridge. Yet, depending on where on the spectrum kiddo is, the consistency of math and reading can be grasped easily. This is when we think that kiddo has amazing faculties, but these very aptitudes are a sign that conceptual inability is real because when asked to tell what the story or the moral of the book is, he can't answer that question.

By the time kiddo becomes a teenager, all or some of the efforts lavished on him to teach him academically and learn about life, have in some ways become counterproductive. At first, as a kiddo, he tried, really did, because time brought some contextual facets to his life and some feelings of what is needed to be done but without concept it just does not make sense, it does not stick. All the repetitions are beyond tiring now, the efforts in all these areas are overwhelming, he just cannot understand them all and they trigger anger. It is exhaustive. He still wants to please the parents, he really wants to badly, but it is just too much. He can't, it has always triggered irritability but now, it is impossible to overstate how difficult it has always been. This effort must come to an end.

Now, well into teen, the battle has ended, there is no more fighting, mom and dad understand he is better with less pressure. There is peace in the house. In some way, since then he is making small progress. It is what it is.

Depending on how much context Junior can grasp, he is able to do certain things. He might be able to work, make the most wonderful expresso each time and will greet people with enthusiasm. Reading Donald Tripett, the so called "case 1" obituary, we find out he was eventually able to drive and hold a job as a bookkeeper but remained with obsessive behaviors and mechanical speech.

While most of this deep dive into what it is like to live with autism from being a baby into adulthood, there is a point to be made for some level 1 individuals on the spectrum because their suffering is not to be minimized. Although many will always wonder what it could be like to connect fully, to understand social cues, facial expression and be totally accepted, it remains that having autism is a very limiting way of living.

CHAPTER 5

The Logic of 75 Common Symptoms of Autism

The following list of symptoms is never mentioned on the NIH website or any other official descriptions of ASD, let alone within any definition of autism, yet many of these symptoms are present in nearly all cases. Officially, it is as if they don't exist. They are not considered actual symptoms of autism, but rather individual unexplainable issues seen more as behavioral than actual indicators of autism. Such "omission" is a direct result of not having a definition of autism; it makes a tacit nod to the long surviving, hard to get rid of beliefs that parental incompetence is part of this illness. It is disheartening to witness parents left with no alternative but to address the challenging symptomatology of their children, such as poop smearing, using behavioral therapy methods that were never intended to address such issues, and additionally resort to speech therapy when the child struggles with pronoun recognition. A lack of understanding and comprehension of autism lead to broken, compartmentalized, disjointed and ineffective treatments.

One can understand that for those who are of the opinion that autism can only be treated with therapies: ABA, speech, occupational therapy (O.T), and medications etc. it is impossible for them to believe that there can be one whole encompassing approach.

It is precisely why autism can be understood as a whole, that so much can be done for it. This is the result of many years of meditation, reflections and as mentioned earlier in this book, having taken a different starting point than others.

Many years ago, I realized some prominent symptoms of autism were not as senseless or irrational as people make them out to be. As you will see, many symptoms are just exaggerations of natural movements we commonly make. That said, most of this chapter's logic came since unlocking conceptual inability.

There are essentially three sources for all these symptoms.

- Conceptual inability
- "Stage 12" detailed in a later chapter
- "Phase 7" also detailed in a later chapter.

If you are thinking of someone while reading the explanations of these symptom, given that ASD is a spectrum of difficulties according to Conceptual Inability, you will need to adjust the cursor in your mind to fit the frequency and intensity of the individual you are thinking about. Nonetheless, the reason for the symptom does not change.

At some point in the future, once conceptual inability is accepted, the next step will be to have far more accurate diagnosis with each of the following symptoms graded and classified. No longer will these symptoms be swept under the rug as if they don' exist, they will be part of an all-encompassing far more effective system in relieving suffering.

1: HUMMING

This is probably the most common symptom of ASD. While most symptoms' logic is simple, this is one takes a two steps process to elucidate.

First, we need to understand how the brain feels. The most colloquial way of describing the sensation in the ASD brain is that it feels "scrambled".

That feeling, reported by parents through the "surrogacy method" and recovered individuals on the spectrum is especially pronounced at the top of the head. The feeling inside the head is that the thinking process is scrambled, information gets lost, it does not come through; that creates a feeling of being stuck in place with a total absence of clarity. This is a constant feeling, it never leaves. Humming is meant to alleviate the 'scrambled" feeling that the thinking process is arrested. We can compare it to when we forget a word and hum for a few seconds in the attempt to recover the word we are looking for. We instinctively hum to unlock whatever process we feel is hindered. The process is exactly the same for people on the spectrum, except that the feeling is constant in all facets of thinking. This is one the many reasons why 25 years ago, I declared autism to be a painful illness. Imagine for a second to live with such a feeling 24/7.

2: SPINNING
Spinning is a way of losing or detaching oneself from the agony of living with ASD. Unlike laughing that is a non-voluntary symptom, spinning is voluntary. It seems as if spinning is more of a level 2 ASD than level 3. One needs to have a sense of not connecting to alleviate the feeling, whereas level 3 does not have any sense of connection and does not feel he is failing at connecting. Spinning is an attempt at catching up with the disconnect. It works at reconnecting for a few seconds to a few minutes and then needs to be repeated.

3: LAUGHING
According to the remedies that improve the "totality" of autism, (See Symptom "Tiptoe" and "Aggravated by sound" for a more complete definition of totality) laughing seems to happen when the patient is very stressed. Laughing is not a behavioral choice. It is just the nature of the person that makes laughing occur in inappropriate situation. The driver for the laughter is the stress generated by being on the spectrum and the suffering that occurs due to that. It is like an endorphin reaction. In the neuro typical (NT) population this situation can occur during a sustained effort such as running a marathon. The effort is so intense that it triggers laughing as a coping mechanism to the pain. The stress of autism is constant; hence the laughing is inappropriate most of the time.

Laughing also seems to relate to the effect of being alone. People who spend extended amounts of time, months to even years, develop immoderate laughter. Biomed talks about yeast overgrowth as if it were making the child behave in a drunken manner. Antifungal medication is prescribed rarely to any avail because the problem is not yeast which, due to law of adaptation, will regrow anyway.

4: NO SPEECH

Given conceptual inability, speech is impossible to understand or make sense of what is heard. It is gibberish to the ear, just like it sounds "gibberish" to the parents. The children repeat sounds they hear much like we repeat the sounds we hear when we try to sing a song in a foreign language, without any idea what the lyrics are. Interestingly, I have asked parents to try to understand the sounds rather than words, in many cases suddenly they hear words and soon, by noting the sounds they realized that the child was speaking as if all the words were attached as one word.

5: NO EYE CONTACT

People are not seen as people but rather as objects. Who has eye contact with a table or a vase? Being seen as an object rather than a person, is the feeling many parents have when their child looks at them. There is no comprehension of the subtleties in other people's eyes either. Eye contact is difficult, not because it is as much as there no purpose for it. Eye contact also requires understanding of what the other person is trying to convey. Conceptual inability prevents understanding. On milder level of autism, difficulty with eye contact is as if there is a veil before the eyes, emblematic of the autism "bubble" so many speak of.

6: NO SOCIAL CONTACT

Much like lack of eye contact and speech, social contact is only possible according to how much and how deep the inability the child has. None of these can function without ability. It is autism. Without ability people are seen as object. In fact, an object, a red cube is more important than the mother since the mother is an object that moves, makes sounds, comes close, sometimes yells, forces me to do things (I don't understand), the cube is better, I can hold it, keep it and bite it if I want, it does not do anything to me, but no hard feelings please.

7: ANGER WITH A DROP OF WATER ON THE SHIRT
This might be the first symptom I elucidated, and it is definitely the one that gave momentum to understanding autism as a whole. A drop of water is seen as a fact. It is not understood as something that will dry and will disappear in a few minutes. It is a forever stain. As the mind is at a standstill, scrambled, the concept that the drop will dry does not exist and even once dried, it is still seen as there. It is a fact; the shirt must be changed. There is no alternative to this. The shirt is stained forever, it must be changed come hell or high water.

8: LINING THINGS UP
This is a stage 12 symptom reflecting its cardinal characteristics: Order and perfection, or more precisely for stage 12; Overcontrol. It is a way of finding resonance within because the body and everything else in life feel so chaotic. Lining things up is a way of reconnecting with some very basic internal elements to find control through order.

9: LACK OF FEAR
Yes, no concept of fear equals no fear. I understand it is redundant to say and by now it seems obvious but there is nothing simple when raising a child on the spectrum. I have seen many parents take turn to go out to the store because they could not go outside with their child as it is too dangerous. The time devoted to cope with such symptom is just too great to fully understand the dedication needed on the part of the parents. Taking the child, even with a harness is too dangerous, He can bolt out onto the parking lot and the street without any thought of danger at all.

10: PRONOUNS
The National Autism Association talks about "reversing pronouns". That is not accurate. It is a function of not knowing who "me" is, in addition to not recognizing others. In many cases the problems start with "me" on the physical level as in the feeling that not even the body itself is put together. One leg is floating here, and an arm is floating there. Before

learning "me" and "others", all these parts of "me" must be gathered and put together. Little can be expected from the scattered child under these conditions, trying to teach anything will be wasted time and anxiety generating training.

11: TENSING
Tensing is not dissimilar to flapping is a form of gathering energy built up in the body, concentrating it and then release it for a momentary feeling of calm or relaxation.

12: SHAKING OR FLAPPING HANDS
Shaking of the hand is a function of needing to focus. Without it can't focus. It is like Tom cruise needing his bat to think. The feeling is less intense than flapping. It is not so much excitement as it appears but rather shaking off the excess to be able to have attention. "I want to play so I shake. If I don't, I can't play or see or focus at all on anything.

13: TURNING LIGHTS ON AND OFF
The same holds true for opening and closing drawers. It is a simple function of concept and context of what she can make happen that autistic individual lack so much of. This is combined with the mesmerizing effect of repetitive action. It is the same as looking at a piece of lint or a string.

14: REPEATS QUESTIONS
"Did you go to the playground?" "Go playground" Repetition is simple in the sense that it does not require creating an answer. There is no comprehension of what is asked, an answer is a world away from his capacity to express anything that resemble a comprehensive answer.

15: SPEAKS ONLY OF HIS INTERESTS
The only thing that is real is what she speaks about. This is generally seen in level 1 or mild autism since there is actual speech. The conceptual inability is not 100%, it allows some capacity for only one subject. That one thing or subject is the only thing that exists, that is why they are so adamant to speak about it. There is nothing else within her reality, how could anyone not be interested? Inability cannot transform into full tilt

ability without treatment although the subject can change. Interestingly, I have noticed that when a change of subject happens the previous one seems to be lost. One interest does not really build another, rather one is forgotten and is replaced by another.

16: HANDWRITING DIFFICULTY

A letter is meant to be a fluid concept that flows from one letter to another to make a word. In cases of autism, the letters are broken down into small bits. The first time I observed this was truly a Eureka moment. I was looking at what was supposed to be an "A". What I actually saw was: two slanted, slightly wiggled lines not meeting at the top and a transverse line cutting through the two vertical lines near the top. I realized then, after looking at hundreds of these that the child was not writing an "A". An "A" was what everyone thought it was but to the child it was just three lines that he was taught to draw on a piece of paper. What I realized was that he had broken the letter down, into three lines because he was told to do it. In his mind, it was three lines and not an "A". The same pattern held with all the other letters as well. An "e" was written like an upside-down Nike Swoosh and at the end of the swoosh was a small, downward pointing dash rather than one curving motion. He has broken the "e" down, into two components, a swoosh, and a dash but he had no knowledge of the letter "e" itself. Truly, a eureka moment as I saw the same pattern repeat for most letters. I also realized that for every approximation we think he has written he receives encouragement for a wiggly line which is counterproductive.

17: SMELLING OF HAIR

This is the last symptom I was able to make sense of, as it really baffled me to no end. Most of the time they seem to smell the hair. Some parents have assumed that it is because of the different shampoo between father and mother but others said they use the same shampoo, but the child does not smell the father's hair. So, it was a mystery until I realized that it has to do with phase 7, that of feeling rejection. It is common for women to cut their hair after giving birth, or after the children have left the home. When a woman cuts her hair after giving birth it is a sign of needing to reclaim some independence in life. In nature we see the hedgehog turn her back on the babies and expose her spikes to stop breastfeeding, the opposite feeling of lusciousness chocolate gives. When children on the spectrum have an obsession to smell the hair it is generally when it is long. Long hair gives the child a feeling of acceptance, it relieves the prominent feeling of rejection. I wonder if it wouldn't be a good thing to have kids on the spectrum keep long hair as well.

18: DIFFICULTY POTTY TRAINING

This is far more a matter of integrity rather than G.I. Tract problems solved with probiotics and magnesium. While some supplements can help, they are not what is at issue here. At issue is "I need everything I have; I don't know what will happen if I lose something". Passing stool is like losing a part of oneself. Quite often these kids cause their own constipation. This is why they have difficulty getting potty trained, it is also why parents who particularly sensitive speaking of the child "Withholding". The body is giving severe physical signals to poop and yet they fight it with all their might to prevent the feeling of loss. Passing stool is lived as a loss of body integrity, it is like losing a leg. Over time they may learn to poop in the diaper as it is not a total loss or may want to keep it in the closet as is often the case. Incidentally, by conjecture, this is why the kids don't like the flushing sound as they know that with that sound the poop is gone and lost.

19: READING CREDITS

Completely logical. A movie is a series of moving and talking images full of emotions. It does not get more conceptual than that. Comparatively, reading credits or watching traffic videos online is factual and simple. FUN!

20: REWINDING YOUTUBE VIDEOS EVERY FEW SECOND

The rewinding of videos or movies to specific moments is to capture the moment of little connection their inability allows them to make with their personal affinity. That moment, different in every child, is a moment of resonance. It can only be limited, and the limitation can only be according to how much conceptual ability the child has, most of the time it is rather short. It is part of stimming, it relieves stress.

21: SPINNING WHEELS

This is often one of the first symptom to be noticed by the parents. The fire truck is laying on its side in the living-room and instead of putting it right side up, the ASD patient spins the wheels. Little do we know that he has no idea the truck, is a truck. This is like reading the credits at the end of a movie, only the wheels make sense. There is a slight mesmerizing effect, perhaps like the credits or the short video clips but it is the straightforward simplicity of the action that fits the limited conceptual inability.

22: PLAYING WITH WIRES AND DUST BALLS

I spoke about this symptom in the earlier chapter "The autism experience". Without conceptual ability a dust ball or a wire found on the floor are the equivalent of a toy truck. In fact, given conceptual inability a string is far more attractive than a toy truck.

23: CAN'T EXPLAIN THE MORAL OF THE STORY

Yes, absolutely, that makes total sense. Remember "reading credits", just factual. The moral of the story is a human concept. The only concept that an individual on the spectrum senses in a guttural way is injustice expressed by crying, screaming, throwing things. It is a very physical basic reaction, the moral of the story requires formulating thought to be expressed through the mouth that is too out of reach to an individual on the spectrum.

24: LIMITED FOODS

Conceptual inability precludes the sense of discovery. There is no world. Under such general experience who needs more than one food? There is no need! One or two foods is enough, there is no sense in eating anything else. One or two foods give a sense of consistency so needed to cope with ASD. More foods are very confusing.

25: NOT CARING WHEN OTHERS TAKE TOYS

This is most often seen in level 3 cases. The child does not care whether something is taken away from him even when it is snatched from his own hand, she does not react. Conceptual ability in these cases is seriously compromised. This is a child who might be happy with a piece of string.

Attachment does not exist. In such a case, a sign of the child getting better is actually reacting with anger when something is taken away from her.

26: HOLDING ON TO TOYS

Holding a toy is a security. It is like "Wilson" in the Tom Hanks movie "Castaway". It is a connection. Most parents would like it to be a doll or a truck, however it is often a soft plastic cube often used to chew to relieve pressure in the teeth.

27: PRESSING THE EYES

When there is pain in cases of autism, pressure generally relieves. The "squeeze machine" was invented for that reason. When it comes to the eye, there can be no doubt the pressure they apply is real. Sometimes one can see the finger so deeply sunk into the eyeball that we can literally feel the depth of his pain. Amelioration by pressure is what we, in homeopathy, call a Generalized symptom. Pressure ameliorates the pains, but one should not be naïve, while relieving pain is great, so much pressure is applied, there isn't any doubt that damage is being done to the eyeball. Do note, that paradoxically, while pressure generally helps, a hug will not be as welcome as one might thing. During a hug one does not have control of when the hug will be released, a stage 12 matter.

28: PRESSING IN THE BACK OF THE EAR

This is an interesting symptom that used to be more common than it is today. A sidebar: Over the years, a few symptoms I used to see frequently, diarrhea or pressing the back of the ear, I don't see as often as I used to. I try to not fall in the "pain" category. If I were to settle for this kind of elementary "explanation" I would never have arrived at the rock bottom definition of autism exposed in this book.

29: RUNNING ALL OVER THE PLACE

There are several reasons for running or pacing throughout the house. It is very common to have children run and crash into the couch to relieve physical G.I. tract pain. One other reason for running is due to an unrelenting buzzing feeling in the body as if there were electricity coursing through the body. The same is true in the brain, in which case, if it is strong enough, it leads to banging of the head.

30: CONSTIPATION

This is less a function of G.I. tract issues such as yeast, gut bacteria etc. and far more an issue of holding on. Holding or more appropriately "Withholding" is a defensive issue. I can't let go. Do refer to "Difficulty potty training". Losing poop is physical, it is a thing, not an idea or a need, that is the difference.

31: AGGRAVATED BY BABY CRYING

This symptom is driven by a deep desire to have order (Stage 12). A crying baby is perceived as if something wrong going on. Yes, there is the sensitivity to that sound too, but the sensitivity is triggered by the sentiment that there is something wrong and that it needs to be fixed. The feeling is also augmented in level 1 or 2 ASD by the sensibility to injustice. As such, a level 1 individual on the spectrum might want to check what is happening with the crying baby, which is an oddity; if she notices that a parent is being harsh to the baby then she will have what will be interpreted as a tantrum but in actuality, it is an emotional outburst to injustice.

32: AGGRAVATED BY SOUNDS

Sounds are difficult to process due to the buzzing nature of a travelling sound wave. It goes straight to the brain and increases the buzzing, augmenting the scrambled sensation already there. In this situation the only thing one can do is cover the ears. While an ASD patient is demanding through his strong inclination of having tantrums, one should know that the symptoms themselves are experienced as demanding and burdensome on him as well.

33: AGGRAVATED BY RUNNING KIDS

Running kids are nearly by definition; disorderly. Several factors come into play in this instance. There is no way to tell what is going on. A kid is going here, another kid is going there, they are screaming and laughing, it's all contrary, there is no sense. nothing jives. Chase is different, it makes sense. All run this way or that way, that is OK, like a flock of birds, though a lot of ASD kids don't understand they should alternate between chasing and being chased. Chase is deeply instinctual; I think that is why most ASD kids "play" chase. It is the reason I don't take it into consideration as social improvement.

34: HANDLING GENITALS

Much like chasing is instinctual there is something similar with the handling of genitals. It is not unusual to have very young kids to be stimulated by the presence of a female in the room. It is also common to have ASD boys choose to parallel play with a girl, not be aroused while having no interest in anyone else. The attraction for the opposite sex is common for boys, I am not so sure it is there for girls. Handling genitals is however different. Given the few dozen remedies listed with the behavior, most of them have handling of genitals due to a physical sensation, burning, drawn sensation etc. only two remedies are for the pleasure of it.

35: TIP TOE

I don't hear about this symptom as frequently as I used to. We could say that the reason for tiptoeing is because of pain but I am quite skeptical of linear thinking because we can make anything up and sound good. I prefer to understand the logic of symptoms through the experience. There is widespread low muscle tone concomitant to ASD, which is why most kids go to physical therapy. Low muscle tone fits with conceptual inability in the sense that it is partly due to exhaustion. In homeopathy we like to analyze cases in terms of "totality" that represents one seamless, logical whole. We don't pick a remedy for one symptom and another remedy for another symptom, that is a very amateurish and potentially dangerous way of approaching these cases, yet so often seen nowadays. Exhaustion on the mental level should be reflected in some way on the physical and emotional level, that is totality. This is what has been so systematically successful for me rather than randomized remedies for specific symptoms, which will never return neuro-typical behavior.

36: ROUTINE

This is the opposite of changes. As the saying goes "I don't have to think about it". No surprises, no need for outbursts. Given the overtaxed body, routine is easy. It makes life livable. The more routine the better, it prevents stress. Most parents program every day of the week as a compensatory process to avoid outburst and more typical behavior however it gives false sense of well-being, on the other hand it keeps the house relatively quiet.

37: AGGRAVATED BY CHANGES

Changes are disruptive, as adaptation itself requires a process that conceptual inability leaves little room for. Anything can go wrong, and control can be lost at any time. Even a small change contains the potential of a million things going wrong. From that point of sensation, the feeling is "I will fight to prevent anything out of the ordinary". Changes are the exact opposite of what is most sought after: Consistency. With it there is no surprise, nothing will happen I don't know about, and I won't be stressed.

39: NOT PLAYING WITH TOYS APPROPRIATELY

To play with toys, one must see toys as such. Have you ever used something for a purpose other than what the item is intended for and be proud of your solution? It is the same with a toy for a kid on the spectrum. The initiation of play, the appeal of rolling the truck, stop at an imaginary intersection, load it up and unload is nonexistent. There is no concept of a truck, or doll. Spinning the wheels when the truck is on its side, now that is great. It is simply using the truck for another purpose than it is destined for. Spinning the wheels is very basic, seemingly senseless but fun.

40: OBSESSIVE INTERESTS

Obsession is interesting but I am not so sure the word itself is appropriate. Familiarity is the key. It is doing the same thing to feel good, whereas "obsessive" suggests that it is constant without any control of it which, on level 3 ASD is somewhat true. It is like repeating sentences. Those sentences exist in the mind, they feel good, they are comfort. In obsession there is no comfort. With familiarity, I can always go back to them. They don't offer any surprises. "Stage 12" M.O. is to be on a constant alert, ready to fight, surprises are anathema. Repeating the same thing all the time, is not so much refining as a training would be, it is being with something familiar. When I go to a Chinese restaurant I order "Chicken with broccoli and black bean sauce". I never order anything else because of the familiarity, not the obsession, it gives me the comfort that I will like what I am about to eat.

41: ROCKING

This is a sign of frustration and low energy. The child is tired from running back and forth, the only thing left to do is relieve the feeling that the brain is scrambled, sit and rock. The purpose is not so different from people sitting on a rocking chair out on the porch. People ask the child to do tasks, the child has a faint feeling that she should be doing something, but she can't. Everything in life is enormously stressful, all the child can do is sit and rock. The speed and the vehemence are equal to depth of illness.

42: JUMPING

Jumping is much like restless. The physical sensation ASD produces in the body is so uncomfortable that the kiddos must move to relieve the buzzing sensation in the body. They just don't know what to do with their bodies. There is also at times a lightning sensation in the legs or the feet, at other times there are little cramps, banging the feet on the floor relieves that.

43: AGGRAVATED BY CUTTING NAILS OR HAIR

Losing integrity is the in and out of symptoms. Nails and hair are part of the body, the feeling is not that they are getting cut, the feeling is that he is losing them. They will be gone. One would say, well, cut them once and then they'll see that they are still there. That is easy to say when one has conceptual ability or physical integrity but when one does not have that then each time is a new time for losing. This is also made worst by restricting the child to be able to cut safely but then taking control of his body only aggravates the problem. One way of dealing with this is by giving some control to the individual. "You need a haircut, it will take 9 minutes, OK?" If the child has some cognition, he will most likely be fine with it, but not a minute over. Respect that, it is important. Over the years, some of the symptomatology will diminish with repetition, contextually the child accepts it but that does not mean he is feeling safe about the process.

44: REJECTING PHYSICAL CONTACT

Physical contact is very uncomfortable for a lot of ASD individuals. They feel physical contact to be immediately restrictive. It is perceived as a loss of control over their body much like someone is physically controlled by the police. The feeling is that strong and deep especially when there is relentless hyperactivity. Some overly controlling therapists can increase the feeling there is something wrong with him. As such, his feeling is that he has done something wrong.

45: BURROWING UNDER BLANKETS

Burrowing is a symptom I am not fully sure about. Naturally, we think of the blanket providing some weight to help with physical integrity, the dry version of wanting to be in water to restore body integrity or the squeeze machine. I thought it might be that children who liked to burrow under blanket didn't like bath but that has not proved itself to be correct though one does not exclude the other. There is also burrowing between cushions but that is more like a squeeze. So, in the end I have not figured this symptom beyond being similar the relief brought by the squeeze machine.

46: SWINGING

I understand swinging only in terms of repetition, as in routine. It is a more intense activity than rocking. The consistency of the swinging motion is what is so deeply satisfying. It is reliable, nothing can interfere with it, it is always the same until she decides to stop it, there is a sense of control, so important in ASD modus operandi. Rocking has the component of head banging against the cushions that swinging does not have. There is also the element of speed with is incredibly attractive as all kids love swinging anyway but I have seen kids stay on the swing for hours, even as nighttime has come with a big broad smile. Perfect consistency and not a care in the world.

47: INABILITY TO FOCUS

Conceptual inability is the root of the inability to focus. Focus on what? Assuming you are not a chemist, imagine you are at a party, and someone asks you to focus on a board full of chemical formulas. What you are going to do is the exact same thing a kid on the spectrum does, give it 15 seconds and walk away, understanding that chemical formulas have no bearing on the party. No need. It is the same feeling for a child in front of a piece of paper for his homework. It has no purpose or consequences at all for him.

48: NOT RECOGNIZING JOKES

What makes a joke funny is its concept within a context. Since neither truly exist in the mindset of someone on the spectrum, jokes can only be taken at face value. Level 1 autism individuals can acquire some contextual perspective through exposure and life experiences and come to understand some daily contexts, not jokes but at level 3 one is living in a world made only of things or facts. So, the expression "it's raining cats and dogs" constitutes three facts. "raining", "dogs", "cats". It can't happen. There is no concept of analogy or absurdity that it is raining so much beyond belief, saying "raining cats and dogs" does not make sense.

49: FLAT, ROBOTIC VOICE

Our voices reflect emotions but with ASD emotions, beside the ones of action and reaction of Stage 12 emotions are disabled. This is not to say that individuals on the spectrum are psychopaths or sociopaths, that is Stage 17. Far from it, ASD individuals show a lot of empathy as we have seen when a baby is crying, or a sibling gets yelled at. They do not like that at all and often make their feelings known by pushing a parent away or by screaming. The problem with ASD is an inability to process emotions as if the mind is exhausted, it can only deal with a very small finite amount, that is why the voice is robotic. The voice is used only to pass along the most essential information, not more can be done.

50: NOT USING GESTURES

Gestures have meanings, without conceptual ability gestures which generally convey subconscious emotions cannot be accessed. One consistent gesture seen is pushing. They tend to defend their sense of autonomy and the autonomy of others as well.

51: WAKING AT 3 AM

This symptom is interesting and can be explained only by conjecture rather than through conceptual inability, Stage 12, or Phase 7. I went back to the years when I was in Homeopathic School and one of our teachers wanted us to use what he termed, "Mappa Mundi" that was a collection of old and new thoughts of patterns and beliefs from all four corners of the world. I dug up my Mappa Mundi and looked at the 3AM time slot. Interestingly it said, "Detox of blood, recovery and planning". How about that? I thought. Most of the Biomed approaches concentrate on detoxifying procedures. Blood test of heavy metals do seem to suggest that people on the spectrum have a processing/detoxifying problem though some cases do very well with fern remedies which are metallophyte. It is not central to recovery; therefore, only limited improvement following that type of treatment can be expected.

There is an exhaustion aspect to conceptual inability. Children give the appearance of being physically hyper but are mentally exhausted especially when they are forced to understand their surroundings. As such, waking at 3AM makes sense as an interference with the deep process of recovery that is part of a good night sleep.

52: TROUBLE EXPRESSING NEEDS

The needs for level 3 individuals on the spectrum, are at times nearly non-existent. We can track back to pregnancy, and find that feeding, the most basic need of all, appears to be an issue given that *"low birth weight increases the odds of the baby being on the spectrum by 60%"* (NIH). If basic survival is a challenge in utero, followed immediately after birth with difficulties breast feeding, other needs will also rank low. If in fact, there is a genetic issue with autism, it may well be at that Feeding – Gene junction in utero. As far as I tried to explore literature on that aspect of research, it does not seem to be an avenue of interest now. I think looking at the "trouble expressing needs" as a continuum from pregnancy is the best way to look at ASD in perspective and reveal its whole. Naturally, from conceptional inability perspective having trouble expressing needs is a bit of a misnomer as "need" does not really exist.

53: NOT GETTING SIGNALS FROM BODY LANGUAGE, OR TONE OF VOICE

It is important to understand that the mind of individuals on the spectrum is overwhelmed. It can't process much; the glass is already full.

Processing more is not an option. The overall needs are extremely basic, processing subtleties of body language, facial expressions are too complex to the basic state that autism actually is. Have you ever found yourself in the wrong place with a crowd not to your liking? All you want to do is leave. There is no point in figuring out what their purpose is, it is too complicated and won't be of much use for you? That is basically the same for a child on the spectrum. There are too many individual subtleties, one replacing another so quickly it is neither possible, important nor needed to understand.

54: NOT TAKING PART IN "PRETEND PLAY"

Pretend play is a conceptual issue. Without concept there is no play. Return of conceptual play is a good sign of being on the way to recovery. Pretend play is a fantasy, there is no fantasy in the ASD mind, it can mainly deal with simple facts rather than make things up. This meets with the well-known inability of lying for people on the spectrum. They can't make things up. To make things up one also needs to have the sense that he is going to lose something. Losing something, is often not existent as seen when "someone can take something away from him and he won't react".

55: LACK OF COORDINATION

I don't know how to explain this symptom in a meaningful way other than say that stage 12 is best represented by the words, "chaos" and its counterpart "order". The functioning of an ASD body is so chaotic that it's integration in space which requires order is simply not there. Another reason for lack of coordination comes from the exhaustion part of the conceptual inability. Imagine doing any activities, after several sleepless days, for sure you will be staggering to go up and down the stairs for the laundry, dusting with be very randomly done and paying attention to the bills will be complicated. I take tango classes. Last week, I was particularly tired for having burnt the midnight oil on this book. The teacher showed the simplest six steps routine and I just could not process it on the dance floor. I felt I was so bad that I left. The next day, after a good night sleep, I got up, thought about it for a second and there it was, the simplest routine I staggered through the day before. It is impossible to undervalue the exhaustion aspect in autism as it contributes to so many symptoms.

56: IMPULSIVENESS

Impulsiveness is a product of Stage 12 Modus Operandi. It stems from the sense of being suddenly overwhelmed; and the reaction is not to lay down as in Stage 2, but rather to fight or create chaos to get out of the perceived situation.

57: NOT RESPONDING TO HER NAME

There are several reasons for not responding.

1. Lack of comprehension. Remember that speech, without conceptional ability, is only sound. Concept allows for rational thinking to eventually make sense of it. When people are looking at a baby and the sound (not name) 'Joe" comes out of their mouth, baby understands after some time that might "Joe" has something to do with him, and then the baby's process connects the dots, "oh, that is what they call me", and then in fairly short order an internal voice says, "that's my name". In the mind and psyche of a kid on the spectrum that process takes a very long time.
2. ASD "Level 3" does not have much of a "me" concept. Me might be an arm here and a leg there as is described in symptom "needing pressure". It is hard to have a sense of self without the prerequisites that make the whole understood.
3. In this world of forms and things, all there is, is non-sense demand. There is no name, there is no salient reason for turning the head. The head is just full of buzzing sounds incapable of processing anything to a meaningful end.

58: NOT UNDERSTANDING EMOTIONS

It is very difficult for an individual on the spectrum to understand emotions. Over time, some understanding of emotions will come within contextual situations in life. The recognition of emotions will be very basic such as anger when mom raises her voice. Most of the time however, inability is what it is. We, from the outside can't understand how it is possible to not recognize what appears to us so basic and crucial to life. We feel that if emotions can't be recognized the first time around, at least "at some point" with repetition, some form of acknowledgment should happen and yet it does not. This is extremely frustrating; therefore, we must understand inability in the first place and that the necessity of understanding emotions in other people is not something that is needed. Let's say you want to go to Italy; you think learning Italian would be great. But you don't learn the language, not that important, and even if no one speaks your language while you're there, it will still be OK. At worse, you may feel like you missed something. It is the same for the individual on the spectrum except that he does not feel like he has missed much.

59: NOT STRETCHING ARMS OUT TO BE PICKED UP

The ASD individual does not know much about emotions. It is not that he does not have emotions, he does not know about emotions. It is not a narcissist disposition; he just does not know. In fact, I find ASD individual quite emotional and wanting others to be content as I described "Aggravated by crying babies".

60: CROSSING THE STREET WITHOUT LOOKING

Danger is a concept. Driving 200 miles an hour is dangerous for some but not for others. The notion of danger comes from understanding that bad things can happen when doing something dangerous. For a lot of children on the spectrum danger doesn't exist because the notion of dying also does not exist much like the basic need for eating.

61: LIKING BATHS

Most kids on the spectrum love to be in the water, take long baths, at times very cold, other times very hot. What is important is to understand that being in water is an opportunity for them to feel physical integrity as they often feel their body is not put together but rather in pieces. The experience of parts of the body feeling scattered came through the "Surrogacy method" that was the purpose of "One Heart, One Mind". There are several remedies that get rid of this symptom very quickly within the whole state of autism.

62: AGGRESSION

This is a function of the main feature of Stage 12: Fight to prevent the feeling of chaos, disorder and being controlled. Anything that disturbs this fragile state of order triggers overwhelming feelings that must be addressed immediately by aggression. Only aggression is relevant, only aggression restores control.

63: RAGE AT HEARING "NO".

It is also a function of Stage 12 M.O. Fight is central to stage 12. Hearing "No" is an afront. It cannot not be accepted. In the mind of someone on the spectrum, whatever he asks for is felt as being a crucial piece of maintaining order. It is like the finger preventing the dam from collapsing. The military is a good source of examples to describe Stage 12. The soldier does not say "no" to the drill sergeant. "No" would collapse the entire military order. A lot of parents describe the atmosphere in the house as walking on eggshells. "Stage 12", creates that environment. As we will see in the "Stages" chapter, there is a positive and negative side to each one. With autism eventually, a little bit of comprehension with bring some sense of context.

64: LEARNING LANGUAGE OR COUNTING ON THEIR OWN

This is mainly a Level 1 symptom. Putting letters together and counting are very similar in procedure. B + O = Bo.

It will never change. 1 + 1 = 2. That will also never change. Consistency is extremely important to the mind of an ASD person. It does not offer any surprise which is despised much like transition. A transition is riddled with unknown. A letter in a book, does not change, it is a thing much like a number is. Learning how to count or read becomes a matter of computing rather than understanding the meaning of the text. As such, while some can read text well, most have great difficulty understanding the meaning of the text.

65: WITHDRAWN

There is no connection with anything. No concept that people are NOT things. There is little or no concept that those little things dangling above my head on the floormat are somehow fun. A thing is a thing, that's it. Nothing more than that. And people are just about the same. They make noise, they come too close, and it is impossible to process all of this because the brain is exhausted or scrambled. Just want to kick the shoes off; actually, take the clothes off and watch TV.

66: RESISTING CUDDLING
The resistance to cuddling is due to Stage 12 as a control issue. They don't want to be controlled in any way unless it is under their term. If they seek cuddling, then it is OK but cuddling them is felt like an imposition upon their restless bodies.

67: DOES NOT UNDERSTAND SIMPLE QUESTIONS
What we consider simple is not simple to a child on the spectrum. If it were, she would do it. The problem is not being able to answer the question because the question itself does not make sense.

68: HEAD BANGING – SELF HARM
Most of the time we feel the child suffers from headaches but that is not so true. The feeling is that the brain does not work, it should but it does not. As such it is a physical experience much like when we don't remember a word and we lightly pound our foreheads with our hand or fist. That is the feeling here except that the problem is not about remembering one word but rather not getting this brain to function and not remembering any word. There are two main areas where function feel like it is not happening. The frontal cortex and top of the head. The frontal cortex feels like it is stuck, like a rusty screw whereas the top of the head feels like scrambled eggs; instead of orderly routing, the feeling is that information is only going around nonstop not finding a final point of expression. There may be another phenomenon in action. At times inflicting physical pain to oneself is better than experiencing emotional agony. This is a thought that has recently entered my mind, I feel it is worth, exploring.

69: MELTDOWN
Meltdowns are a function of Stage 12. They are the way for ASD individuals to gain control. The phrase "my way or the highway" relates well to Stage 12. They must have what they want, it is a matter of order, survival and keeping integrity. It does not have to be a thing. Taking a different

road, going in a store, just leaving the house, going to bed, anything can potentially alter what is seen in them as order or incoming disorder.

70: UNRELATED ANSWERS

This situation happens mainly after having had a significant amount of speech therapy. The child has learned and "canned" answers. The question asked is not understood but he has a sense that from the intonation he is supposed to answer something. At that point he "responds" with the learned and retained "answer". It is only with an enormous amount of training that answers are categorized and pulled out when needed. Ms. Temple speaks to that. She is an extraordinary example of this process. She can carry on conversations seemingly flawlessly, but she explains that she retrieves answers that are already there in her mind, the image she gives is in the form of drawers. This may be because Ms. Temple has learned contextually rather than conceptually, but what an absolutely brilliant mind and example though it is not what I seek to achieve with homeopathy.

71: EXTREME PHOBIAS

What will happen if I go in there? The state of being on the spectrum is precarious, on edge, with a deep desire to keep things in order. Entering an unknown space is dangerous. I have taken examples of the military to describe some symptoms, it can apply here again. Extreme phobias stem from the feeling of extreme danger, it is like soldiers entering a city at war. All reasoning tells you to keep out. There is potential chaos here and taking this just one step is too dangerous, I might have to fight. Why go in a situation that can upset order. The intensity of the phobias is generally on par to the reaction. This is opposite of "lack of fear" of course which is conceptual inability dominant whereas "extreme phobias" is Stage 12 dominant.

72: NEEDING COMPRESSION

This symptom seems to come from a sensation that the body needs pressure to feel real. I have seen many cases when the sensation is that the body is falling apart, as if there is an arm floating over here and a leg over there. Pressure on the body seems the bring back a sense of integrity as if putting it back together as a whole. The main remedy with this sensation is Baptisia.

73: SMEARING POOP ON THE WALL

This symptom is mainly seen for level 3 autism but as with everything regarding autism we can't classify this symptom only on level 3. Poop is a thing. We instinctively stay away from substances that don't smell nice to us, but poop is something different. No one likes someone else's poop. But we commonly like our own. With ASD, there is no conceptual sense that it is dirty and disgusting. It is at the top of severity of ASD symptoms. There is zero concept at all, hence no rational thinking. The smell does not bother, no concept there. It is "me" for an ASD child. The feeling is literally, "Look mom, I made a painting". In fact, it is not all that dissimilar to hand painting except that for the parents it is desperately horrendous to live with it and in fact, it is not uncommon for parent to not even mention it.

74: TAPPING ON SOMETHING

Tapping on something is a reminder of being connected to oneself. It is like the bell at the end of a meditation. Most of us do it from time to time, just not all the time. The intensity and frequency of tapping gives an indication of how disconnected to oneself the child feels from his body.

75: RAGE AT DISRUPTING LINED UP OBJECTS

Some children on the spectrum have a strong attachment to order. In such case, lining things up is an attempt at controlling (stage 12), create order and compensate for their lack of concept. Without Within the bounds of order there is some semblance of meaning and control in my life. Lining toys up is an attempt at gaining control through order. It feels good. Stepping out of routine means stepping into chaos again and that is intolerable. Changing a different route to go from point A to Z is unacceptable because it can only bring chaos and challenges.

CHAPTER 6

Choose Homeopathy for Your Child on the Spectrum

Many studies (1) have determined the efficacy of homeopathy in the treatment of autism. *"In 1998, the Spandan institute conducted a study of 54 cases of autism supported by the AYUSH department, of the Ministry of health and Family Welfare, Government of India. The study comprised a case series of 54 children registered, studied and managed at Spandan, during July 1998 to June 2003, suffering from autism spectrum disorder. The findings were as follows:*

- *72% of cases who continued treatment for more than six months showed significant improvement in following order*
  - o *Hyperactive behavior like restlessness and tantrums*
  - o *Impaired sensory defenses*
  - o *Eye contact*
  - o *Speech.*
- *60% of cases with mild autism regained speech*
- *50% of cases (without significant retardation), which continued for more than two years got rehabilitated in mainstream school or slow learners' setup while others were enrolled in Special School*
- *Obsessive acts and self-stimulations showed insignificant change in first six months and took longer to respond".*

"This study demonstrated modifications in the behavior of autistic children as well as improvement in sensory impairment thus reducing autistic features. The findings were encouraging to undertake a systematic study. A specific study was undertaken with following objectives."

"From October 2006 to September 2009, the institute conducted a study of 60 cases of autism. The proposal was submitted to the institutional ethics committee along with comprehensive safety measures."

"The diagnosis of childhood autism disorder was made conjointly by homoeopathic physicians (PMB, PO), clinical psychologist, neurologist and psychiatrist.

Diagnostic parameters were essentially DSM-IV; an autistic child presents with varying degree of cognitive ability. This was assessed by SQ (Social Quotient) through Vineland Social Maturity Scale.

Additionally, EEG, BERA (Brainstem-Evoked Response Audiometry), audiometry, serum serotonin, and genetic karyotyping were carried out at the time of enrollment. Serum serotonin was repeated at the end of the study. According to previous reports, serum serotonin levels were often but not always elevated in autistic children. Therefore, we examined any possible linkage."

1. Barvalia PM, Oza PM, Daftary AH, Patil VS, Agarwal VS, Mehta AR. Effectiveness of homoeopathic therapeutics in the management of childhood autism disorder. Indian J Res Homoeopathy 2014; 8:147-59

The study was extremely well-conducted, and no scientific method of measurement was left aside. *"At one-year post-treatment 88.34% of the patients had improved, 8.33% experienced status quo while only 3.33% had worsened"*. *"The study demonstrated the usefulness of homeopathic treatment with "significant reduction of hyperactivity, behavioral dysfunction, sensory impairment as well as communication difficulty. This was demonstrated well in psychosocial adaptation of autistic children"*.

The first interesting finding is that the percentages are very similar to what I see in my practice although my choice of remedies is far broader than these studies, as they were limited to four remedies. My expectations are far deeper than these studies seek to prove. In my practice, I don't just seek improvements, I absolutely cannot do that, I focus on a process that leads to full reversal, neuro-typical functioning rather than just improvements. My focus is on using homeopathic remedies to restore conceptual ability that unlock eye contact, interaction and speech, indeed full neuro-typical development.

The study was conducted in India within the "AYUSH" department of health. AYUSH is responsible for developing education, research, and propagation in alternatives such as Ayurveda, Yoga, Unani, Siddha and Homeopathy. While the monolithic, closed minded, know-it-all western allopathic medical establishment keeps on criticizing and impeding anything that is contrary to their dictum, homeopaths and others relieve patients of daily suffering. The medical establishment makes basically two types of mind-blowing broad assertions:

1. We know and if we don't know there is no way you can.
2. The assertions we make today will probably change tomorrow.

The first assertion overwhelms the entire discussion. In fact, when the doctor says "nothing can be done" it is largely taken at face value by the parents. What else can one think when the dialogue is so brutally obstructed and deprived of any other voice? To be sure any establishment be it medical or otherwise controls the dialogue with greater or lesser authoritarian tools and methods. In the case of the medical establishment, it achieves much of its promotion under the veil of science for the "greater human good" and spends lot of money to varnish that image.

When the establishment argues that the insignificant amount of money spent on homeopathy and other alternatives should be spent on research keep this in mind these two figures. $2.2 Trillions is spent per year on medical R & D. This astronomical amount is largely supported by the taxpayers. In addition to R & D, $8.3 Trillion is spent on healthcare itself. These numbers need to be compared to $6.2 Billion homeopathic market in its entirety. We are comparing trillions with a handful of billions. Words sometimes don't create the true visual. Here is a different way of looking at it.

Medicine as we know it.

$10.5 trillions: $10 500 000 000 000

Homeopathy total expenditure

$6.2 billions: $- - - - 6 200 000 000

This a difference of $1044 billions!

The second assertion is contradictory to the first, but a little inconsistency is not much of a problem when one controls 100% of the conversation. It is a fact that the medical establishment spends a considerable amount of energy to bombard us endlessly with messages praising its advances. The catch is that it promises us more advances as long as we keep oiling the gears of their machinery. The system is monolithic, it only includes their way of thinking; To its credit, India with its multiplicity of problems has chosen to broaden its medical solutions and make homeopathy the guiding light of the alternative research.

Given the overwhelming dominance of allopathic, western model of medicine around the world one would never know that there are thousands of well conducted homeopathic studies beside the ones noted above that demonstrate homeopathy's effectiveness. There is also a huge body of information coming from practices from around the world where children and adults receiving good care improve just as substantially as these studies suggest. In my practice alone most children improve measurably, to neuro typical. The cases in this book and my previous one "One Heart, One Mind" are a testament to that assertion.

When a singular way of thinking such as medicine as we know it, so overwhelmingly dominates the subject, society loses the benefits of competition of ideas. Entrenched powers are always prejudicial, throughout different societies they have always been and have each time been the falling grâce. The result is that we all lose and suffering, I repeat, SUFFERING continues. The film "Just One Drop" by Laurel Chiten, is a perfect exposé of prejudice, powers and ultimately fraud by the very people who are supposed to remain unbiased in the name of science. Homeopathy stirs a lot of feelings and opinions, to a large part because it is so exceptionally effective, it paradoxically scares the very people it is meant to awe.

What makes homeopathic remedies so effective is the homeopathic approach to illness. A homeopathic remedy by itself has no effect, it is only the accuracy of the remedy for the patient that makes it effective. That explains why we can't give "a remedy for autism" or that taking a remedy can have no effect.

Traditional medicine looks for an external agent such as a microbe, a parasite, or a virus as the cause of disease. The inventions of antibiotics, anti-parasitic and antiviral medication although flawed as we can see with proliferation of antibiotic resistant organisms have done much to advance their cause, but today we are seeing the boomerang effect of their flawed philosophy.

When the disease cause is not accepted to be an invading agent, allopathic medicine looks at intercellular functioning, and recently gene disfunction to try to counter its effects. This is an exceedingly complex undertaking, most particularly so when we take into consideration that our minds and experiences also have an overall effect over the functioning of our bodies, so much so we had to invent the term "placebo effect" to assimilate its influences. Boring into microscopic and trying to interfere with billions of nano second molecular process requires the kind of medical infrastructure that is advocated to us daily. The experience of symptoms is acknowledged as far as it tells the doctor that something is wrong and when the disappearance of said symptoms has been achieved the patient is declared cured even when the patient still needs to take medication to prevent the reappearance of said symptoms. Indeed, if medication is needed to prevent symptoms from reappearing, then diseased physiological processes are still lurking in the body and beyond the symptoms something more fundamental is still active. While we overwhelmingly adopt this approach to disease there is a different methodology, "homeopathic" just as empirical and fact based as the allopathic model we know.

The homeopathic approach acknowledges that the details of the symptoms as they are experienced are primordial and crucial. What is taken as subjective and set aside by doctors, namely the suffering itself, is taken as objective by homeopaths. A disease is not only a set of factual symptoms, but it is also a living experience. Rather than taking at face value what the patient is saying all physical, emotional, and mental experiences are dissected to the most basic component best explained via examples.

The simplest of all cases: Seasonal allergies.

The patient is asked by the homeopath, to describe his symptoms.

"My nose runs just like water through a faucet. My eyes itch and water all the time which can get so bad I am barely able to keep them open especially in sunlight. The only relief I get is when I splash cold water, not hot on my face, or dunk my whole head in the sink."

"When I have seasonal allergies like this I just want to crawl in bed and not do anything. I get very impatient with anything I have to do."

All these symptoms and experience, AS A WHOLE point to one homeopathic remedy, namely Allium cepa. In fact, most cases of seasonal allergy can be quickly relieved with this remedy.

Another patient suffering of allergies could have said: "My allergies cause my throat to tickle. If I could scratch my throat inside, I would! Instead, I make all kinds of sound to try to clear that itch." "Sometimes it is the palate that itches, sometimes it is the back of my throat". "When it gets really bad, I might have some yellow mucus at which point I noticed I start to think that it is not allergies and I become quite anxious".

The symptoms experienced in this case are very different and yet it is still a seasonal allergy case. The remedy here is not allium cepa, the symptomatology does fit at all. Rather the remedy needed is called, Arundo mauritanica with the keynote of itching most particularly in the back of the throat or palate, but not the skin.

These are the simplest examples one can take to illustrate the way homeopathy works. One can easily recognize the difference of physical symptoms and experiences. From this approach, it makes sense that each case requires its own remedy. Arundo mauritanica can effectively only treat the symptoms of the second case. If the second case takes Allium cepa thinking "well, it is seasonal allergies anyway" nothing will happen. This is the main reason why people say, "homeopathy doesn't work". The homeopathic remedy must match the symptoms.

For both cases the regular doctor gives the same medication to counteract the body's expression, it ignores the specific symptoms as the language of the body. As such, it is not surprising then that it creates side effects such as drowsiness, the feeling of dried-up mucus membrane, headaches and so on. By not following the body's own language, in order to change the functioning of the body the medication must be a poison. The fact is all medications are poisons. If one takes too much one dies, that is the definition of a poison. At times the medication the doctor gives helps but the patient still does not feel well, at that point the patient is told that it is all in his or her head. Rather, what we say, "the remedy is not accurate enough". The symptoms and the experience of the disease must go.

As we saw above the homeopathic remedy must match perfectly the language of the body. If the wrong remedy is given, nothing happens. Since the effectiveness of homeopathy is based on matching the accuracy of symptoms to remedy then very little of medicine is needed to create resonance. There is no need to overwhelm the body, the issue of giving something stronger to annihilate the symptoms like there is with medication is never an issue.

When it comes to autism the level of distinction and details is taken to an extremely high level. Make no mistake about it, autism is by far the most difficult condition to treat. For the homeopath, autism, with its lack of language, and complex physical array of symptoms, was always the greatest difficulty to surmount. Thirty years ago, it was impossible to make sense of much of its symptoms. I was baffled, the remedies I gave were based on very specific single symptom. The goal was to make small advances in the relief of suffering, gain that position and move forward from there but as we have seen that approach does not address autism itself.

As they say, perseverance pays off and one day, twenty years ago circumstances guided me in a direction of far greater depth in case taking of an autism case. That lead to great improvements, the patients finally got substantially better, including complete reversal of the condition with return of speech, sociability, and eye contact. I wrote the book "One Heart, one Mind" to detail the method I call "Surrogacy" and its results.

The method remains an integral part of my practice, it is very good, but one would be remiss to think that just this method alone can solve all of the cases. From my vintage point it was clear that more understanding of the logic of symptoms was needed to resolve more cases. Before I go on explaining what advances I made since "One Heart, One Mind" Let's look at why the "Surrogacy method" is so effective and why some patients did not improve.

CHAPTER 7

Case Taking Consultation

"Taking the case" is the phrase used to describe the interactive process of asking questions regarding what the patient feels and physically experiences from his illness or dis-ease. The initial consultation is generally quite a lengthy process varying between two to three hours, in my practice. Analysis to find a homeopathic remedy capable of lifting the totality of dysfunction, is referred to as the constitutional remedy or "simillinum", comes after the interviewing.

The case taking process involves collecting all the facts, using various tools such as interview, observation, perception, and a thorough history of the patient. During the consultation the homeopath comes to an understanding of the language of the body as expressed through individual feelings, functions, and sensations. We have seen in the two previous examples of seasonal allergy that the language of illness are the symptoms it creates in the body. Illness speaks to us through symptoms. The skill is to be able to understand the synergy of the symptom's totality. It is the job of the homeopath to understand the totality of the symptoms in the context of the patient to find a corresponding remedy.

It is the patient who gives an account of his condition, his physical symptoms, and his experience of suffering. This is a departure from the allopathic, material approach, which depends on technology and testing of tissues to find the physical evidence of the disease to treat. If medicine does not find something, you are not ill, "There is nothing wrong with you" regardless of what you are experiencing.

Case taking seeks to understand the disorder expressed and experienced by the person on the physical, emotional, and mental planes. The goal is to enable the patient to describe his internal experience in very fine details to gain a deep understanding of the individual suffering and match that to a remedy.

The initial consultation is a process of very attentive listening and precise questioning to understand the physical symptoms in the context of the whole person, discernable only through the manifestations of the disorder in feelings and functions described by words, gestures and through the senses. Questions follow a thread from the chief complaint to deeper levels of individual unique experience. At a superficial level, the experience of arthritis is common to all, but once we go deeper, individual experiences differ and become nearly endless in every single case. Homeopathy is at its core a deeply individualized medicine. At the deepest level of PEM (Physical, Emotional and Mental), information becomes very individualized. Another example: At a superficial level, a fear of dogs is described by everyone as fear of being bitten. Yet, at a deeper level the fear might have little to do with dogs themselves and more about extreme physical pain in one individual yet may remind another individual of a verbally abusive uncle. In both cases the fear of dog leads to very different directions of physical or emotional pains thereby engendering a very different choice of remedy.

For constipation, as often found in ASC children, the stool can be as hard as a rock, dark pellets that tear the anus; or it can be that the child can go to the potty, even say "it is coming" wiggle on the potty and within a minute lose the desire of going most often by creating a complete constriction of the sphincter muscle to allow the stool to pass. This condition might require an enema after a week though the stool itself is witnessed routinely to be soft. Again, both aspects lead to very different ends and if not investigated properly may lead to the wrong remedy. As we saw in the previous chapter, constipation in children on the spectrum is rarely a function is intestinal flora as is commonly thought though from a practical point of view, until the situation has been resolved might require giving an enema.

The evolution of case taking represents an ever-deepening understanding of how to match "the totality of disease" or states of disorder, to remedies known as "like cures like". Each symptom of a chronic multifaceted disorder acts as a hologram for the entire disorder. The homeopathic principles are of totality, individualization, minimum dose. Individualization often comes with what we call "strange, rare and peculiar" (SRP). One does not pay attention to painful joints in arthritis because it is common in arthritis. If the joint pain is worse after diarrhea (yes, I have seen it) then that becomes an SPR. (Incidentally, the remedy in this case might be *Kali bichromatum*.) Or the joint pain may drive the individual to get up from bed and restlessly pace around. Every time he returns to bed thinking rest will alleviate the pain, the pain returns and so he gets up again. The pain here is combined with a mental symptom of restlessness. The remedy in this case might be *Rhus toxicodendron*, the first remedy I used for myself very successfully. The possibilities of different symptoms are nearly endless. A peculiar symptom for a child on the spectrum might be to not like being in water. The vast majority of ASD patients always want to be in water; therefore, it is common and as such not so interesting just like all arthritis patients have joint pains. Not wanting to bathe become an SRP. To find remedies that match the expression described by the patient we use a combination of symptoms encyclopedias called "Materia Medica" and "Repertories". For example, one can find the remedy Rhus Toxicodendron previously mentioned, in the rubric "Restlessness, which drives him to move from one place to another at night". Similarly, we have in this repertory a rubric "bathing, aggravates". Through experience I have learned which remedies to use in ASD cases.

In addition to this rather straight forward way of taking a case we like to pay attention to spontaneous gestures and irrational, unrelated ad libs. If someone is speaking of a "stabbing pain" and at the same time the spontaneous hand gesture is that of a twisting motion as if wringing a towel, then it is very unlikely that "stabbing pain" is accurate and ought not be considered. Only when speech matches the hand gestures is the information accurate and valuable to take into consideration when choosing a remedy. In consideration of ASD, the challenge is to find a way to take a case for a child who cannot speak.

I refined case taking methodology specifically to overcome ASD innate limitations, perfecting what I call "surrogacy" case taking. Surrogacy is a concept I define as going 'into' the child via an empathic other, most often a parent, with the goal of finding a deep acting remedy. This method evolved specifically in response to the challenges of taking the case of the ASD population. Up until then, the multi-symptomatic nature of the physical presentation, indeed the cognitive deficiencies resulting in poor to non-existent speech and language skills made accuracy impossible. "Surrogacy" case taking broke through the multiplicity of symptoms ASD presents and I was able to bring into focus the deeper individual experience of these young patients.

In essence, "surrogacy" gives voice to a child whose own capacity to communicate is impeded or whose language deficits preclude his capacity to portray physical feelings and emotions with the necessary depth, connection, or self-understanding. "Surrogacy" brings an understanding not just of superficial symptoms and behaviors, but the internal state of the child. From the cases I have seen I have been able to gain an understanding of what the "interior" of autism is rather than make assertions from the outside. It is from that vantage point that, over 25 years ago, I was able to declare that autism is a very painful illness. Again, from this internal vantage point, today I understand why a child wants to poop in his diaper rather than in the toilet. Linear thinking says give pro-biotics, magnesium, or constipation medication. Take your pick, but none of these tell you why the preference of the diaper over the toilet! But first, the process begins with a brief simple questionnaire comprised of nine questions completed by the parents (see appendix). The first three questions are rather straightforward:

1. **What unusual behaviors, interests, obsessions, tastes, aversions, fears - does your child have?**

2. **What makes your child upset or stressed and how does she react when upset?**
3. **What makes her calm, what gives her joy, what is she drawn toward doing, having?**

The answers to these questions are generally very factual, this is where the most common symptoms of ASD are listed. "She spins all day long. She is not able to sit even for a minute to learn how to read". "He laughs without any reason" etc. all super common symptomatology but important to know. Question two is most often answered "He gets upset when we take the iPad away, he can throw things down from the table or roll himself on the floor when we take it away". Again, very common, important to know most particularly at the follow up to monitor progress. Question three answer is commonly shorter than the one for question two.

The child is not present during the consultation. As stated previously, there is not much the child can tell me and, perhaps, I am not the most astute observer. This is possibly a shortcoming, but the main reason I don't see the child is because all the children have gone to so many appointments; they have had to sit as best they could or not, waited or not, been pricked, prodded, patted on the head with a perfunctory smile then shoved into a corner with a couple of ridiculous toys and spoken about in front of them. This is nothing short of horrible in the best of circumstances. In the worse cases, total meltdowns occur, papers fly, things get thrown, tempers flare and embarrassment ensue. I don't see any reason to participate and contribute to this kind of experience. So perhaps observation can give clues, but in my case, I'd rather not cause stress to what is already an extremely stressed child. I ask instead for videos of the child before consultation and then we continue with videos to monitor and witness ongoing changes.

One would think that the observation of behavior during case taking is necessary and useful, but because it is impossible to explore the experience that causes the behavior in a deep way through direct contact with the child, it has limited value. A self-stimulation (stim) is a stim; it is the inner experience of this stim that is meaningful, not so much the outward manifestation of the behavior. It is what animates the stim that is important. Again, the interior is more important than what we see. Given this reality, as we will see, the parents are the solution for this guided exploration.

The second challenge to reach the core of the case is to paradoxically use and yet avoid the multi-systemic, gravely varied and profoundly disturbing symptomology. How does one manage to avoid falling into the vortex of linear symptoms that are so vividly displayed in an ASD case? The obvious gut issues, the high levels of bacteria, fungi, viral agents, the high level of heavy metal toxicity and reach deeper to bring about real changes. How to find totality and logic in this? Make no mistake about it, autism will not be reversed by tackling them directly. This is the approach most parents take and so unfortunately largely fail at. Autism is not due to an infestation of parasites, bacterial infection, or high level of heavy metal. These are only the results of something else in going on in the body. The challenge I must respond to is to keep a bird's eye view of this multi-systemic symptomology to remain unprejudiced to the totality. In this case, prejudice is the lack of understanding of a symptom. Constipation for example has nothing to do with intestinal flora. Even the word constipation is not quite accurate. In most cases, they withhold the action of pooping, as such it is an emotional issue rather than functional, physical issue.

To go beyond the morass of symptom presentation it became clear that I had to find a way to go **far deeper** than the observable and common characteristics of children with ASD. I needed to understand the entire state – *the gestalt* – indeed, the very root or the core of the child's suffering experience. Case taking had to go deeper than noting "flapping" or tantrum behaviors when the child is told "no" but rather be a witness of the internal state of disorder from the very background upon which it is held. This is what "surrogacy" makes possible.

Using this method, individual symptoms are thoroughly described and documented on the physical, mental, and emotional levels and a repertory of indexed symptoms is consulted. A repertory is an index that organizes symptoms. The idea is to find the specific symptom among millions of symptoms in the repertory that lists the remedies that have been proven to heal specific symptom.

When taking the case of a neuro-typical child, the list of complaints is limited and thoroughly discussed. The analysis is uncomplicated, and the totality quickly understood. However, a child on the spectrum presents with a long list of symptoms and behaviors that are not listed even at face value, never mind the interior.

Let's illustrate "repertorization" to arrive at a remedy using constipation, since many ASD children are constipated. The most common stool for a child on the spectrum is that he produces little black pellets like sheep dung, yield. Rubric: "Stool, sheep dung, like." There are forty-one remedies listed in the repertory for this symptom. There is also a rubric called "Stool, balls" where 47 remedies are listed as well as some sub-rubrics for "black", "brown" or 'green" balls. Finding a remedy through such physical symptoms rarely leads to success. Hard, knotty constipation is only a symptom. It does not represent the inner core of the child. It does not give voice to the inner state of the child. One can perhaps affect the "hard knotty stool" with a remedy listed in that rubric, but it does not mean the child's core ASD problem will change unless only by chance. The same can be said about diarrhea, skin issues, or hyperactivity. Too often, parents focus on one problem thinking, "If only my child could go to the bathroom on an every-day basis he would feel more comfortable during the day. I see that he is hurting but if he were not in so much pain, he would be able to focus and he would make progress." While that sounds good and logical in the mind, relieving a local symptom very rarely brings a change in the core.

When the approach is based on a linear, mechanical way of finding a remedy, such as the approach taken by so called sequential homeopathy or CEASE, many different remedies are given in an attempt to affect as many symptoms superficially as possible with the hope of eventually arriving at deep results. Deep results don't happen with superficial remedies. Weeding through the immense array of symptoms is key to reverse ASD.

When it became clear that a different way of accessing the child's deeper state was needed, I began to explore the idea of the "homeopathic genetic tree." This effect has been well documented by contemporary homeopaths in India who often see families living closely together; the same remedy was observed to be effective across several generations with different physical presentations. For example, during the consultation for a child, the mother or grandmother might make a comment such as, "I understand perfectly what he means to say…" or, "I know exactly what my child is going through because when I myself was a child, I had the same feeling he is trying to describe." Such statements can point to a deep and meaningful resonance between individuals. Through such resonance or empathic understanding, the mother can go in detail about what the child is experiencing not because she is the mother but because she happens to be <u>experiencing</u> the symptomatology in a similar way as her child. The wider choice of words from the adult makes the search easier. The effect of this deeper understanding from the part of the parents expands the choice of remedies greatly and leads to more accurate and deeper acting remedies.

Ultimately, this method does not work for ASD because probing feelings and physical pains through the adult family members yield better results only in cases of *organic* illnesses such as asthma, or skin disease, gastro-intestinal issues, auto immune diseases, etc. For autistic children it is nearly impossible to use the immediate arc of relation due to the parent not experiencing autism much beyond, "He is in his own world, and he wants to come out." Parents can accurately relate to the same illness of their child when they have had it themselves, but parents don't have autism before their child, so they are comprehensively at a loss. This challenge had to be overcome.

I started to focus on the pregnancy for the purpose of finding a matching homeopathic remedy; not because something wrong happens during pregnancy but because of the closeness or resonance it brings. When I started to investigate the physical, emotional, and mental planes during pregnancy and chose a remedy accordingly, the results began to improve. In the process, I began to understand pregnancy in a completely different light than what is commonly accepted, and the question became: what is a pregnancy? Autism has indeed really taken me far and wide to find answers consistent enough to make a big difference.

The pregnancy represents a unique opportunity to access the child's inner state. At the level of the Vital Force (VF), a separate state begins its own unique biodynamic being. Although mother and child biologically share a body, one biodynamic state is stronger, over-powers and temporarily replaces the other within the mother. It appears that most of the time, the bio-dynamic state of the child grafts itself onto the mother's Vital Force (VF) 65% of the time. In those cases, the developing biodynamic state is the stronger one and temporarily replaces the biodynamic of the mother. Within the first weeks or months, the state of the child is often stronger simply because it is still connected to "source" which is dynamically more powerful and unincumbered. As this process occurs, the mother is completely taken over by the biodynamic state of the growing fetus; her emotions, physical symptoms and mental state are that of what the child developing inside her, she is no longer herself. This explains, rather poetically I feel, why mothers say things like, "I was not at all myself during my pregnancy". The mom is completely taken over; she is not in her own state any longer but is rather imbued by the state that inhabits her child. Because the change is gradual and it is still, after all, the mother's physical body with which she identifies, she is not aware that she is no longer in her state of prior to pregnancy. From that point on, any experience she describes is descriptive of the child's state, though she is the one experiencing it in all her cells. Everything she feels physically, emotionally, and mentally is that of the child. Sometimes, the switch from one state (mother) to the other (child) is brutal and translates in the morning sickness one feels at the beginning of pregnancy. Unbeknown to herself, she become the reflection of the child. All that is occurring is out of her hand, it is the expression of the growing fetus – the coming child. People who surround the mother also adjust to this new energy with varying levels of difficulties. The mom might think her husband is suddenly behaving differently. That may very well be, the baby is not growing in a vacuum. There are adjustments already being made. She is developing new needs and hubby is like, "wow, what's happening? You used to be so outgoing and now all you want to do is watch TV and get upset if I leave the sponge in the sink instead of putting it away." Who are you? She has become the child! So much essential information is gained from the pregnancy to treat the child.

In the other 35% of pregnancies, the mother's state is the same as the state developing within her. In such instance, since the state is the same as the mother, one can take the present mother's case and find a good remedy for the child.

This deeper, more meaningful understanding happened when a mother said, "she did not feel at all like herself during the pregnancy" and she asked me whether *that* had something to do with her child being autistic. Absolutely not! But that was the beginning of truly understanding autism from the inside. I asked her to describe as much as possible her physical, emotional, and mental state during pregnancy. Through her description during pregnancy, I was able to get substantial homeopathically useable information to prescribe a remedy for the child improved dramatically quickly.

I had reached what seemed like a holy grail of looking through symptoms to see the fundamental expression of the biodynamic state of her child.

The state during pregnancy became crucial to me to find more accurate remedies. I understood that the state during pregnancy is a root upon which I can stand to find a homeopathic remedy. As I asked about the pregnancy in the greatest details possible, searching for the most accurate moments of experience, four of them during pregnancy seem to be more useful:

1. The moment the mother 'knows' she is pregnant. This can be an instinctual feeling. Some mothers know they are pregnant in the moment of conception, literally when the egg is being impregnated with the sperm. The moment is often powerfully ingrained, and the mother can easily go into those feelings at great depth. This has the potential to yield great homeopathically relevant

information, but some caution should be taken as the arousal from intercourse can overwhelm the deeper sensation, and it is usually quite delicate for the mother to talk about.

2. The moment the mother finds out she is pregnant. This is different from the mother knowing she is pregnant. This is commonly the time of taking the pregnancy test. Here, of course, for the purpose of case taking the depth needs to be beyond, "I was excited" or, "I was scared."

3. The entire nine months of pregnancy, especially when they felt **"not at all themselves."** This is definitely the **reflection of the state of the child.**

    "Honey, can you buy a couple of jars of pickles," or, "I want to go to the beach," though it is sub-zero outside. These seemingly meaningless and absurd events are indications of remedies if they reflect in a child who has little sensitivity to cold. I love them because they give such wonderful information. Putting these bits of information together, we can easily recreate the full state and understand it in context. It is so much better to understand pregnancy this way than, "Don't worry, it's your hormones," or, "You'll get over it." It is more of a story than a boring dismissal of chemicals floating around in the body.

4. The delivery. Whether the pregnancy or the delivery is "good or bad," "easy or difficult" does not dictate autism. In fact, no pregnancy or delivery speaks to autism or any other specific disease. Illness and health are not disconnected from each other but rather form a "balance rod." What we know is that some events can create an imprint and that imprint will be a factor in illness. To bring balance back the imprint of the event will need to be erased.

The key is not to interpret pregnancy. An easy delivery can be reflective of an easy pregnancy. "It was so easy, I didn't feel a thing," is commonly considered a positive, but once we scratch the surface it can reflect an "inactive child in utero," "minimal kicking" and little or no effect on the mother, "As if nothing had happened," may reflect a dull state in the child hence become an overarching element in the search of a remedy. The dullness may be reflected in the physical body in the form of *hypotonia* and emotionally dull like "he never cries." Seen that way, "dullness" becomes a crucial piece of information and most likely reflects a central issue on all levels. When a feature such as "dullness" presents at different levels and in different way, it then affords us a branch to hold on to for going deeper into the characterizing aspects of the dullness. I remember a mother speaking about her "easy pregnancy". When she mentioned it to her doctor or family members, she was told to "Just be happy that it's like that." She stopped thinking about it but kept on having a nagging feeling, "I knew something was not quite right." It turned out that one of the most prominent qualities of the child was his dullness. The opposite – or any other configuration - can be true as well. A flamboyant state can echo a hyperactive child, "climbing on furniture," or "waking at 3AM and not needing any more sleep for the rest of the day." I must ask the questions that come to my mind and listen to the answers. One thing leads to another, without the questions we can't have personalization. Anything is possible and needs to be investigated deeply to precisely find the characterizing nature. "Dull" or "hyperactive" are qualities that can lead us deeper into the core but alone don't present enough information to be of value. Questions are pursued focusing on one of these four pregnancy moments to obtain a deeper understanding depending on WHAT and HOW the mother says.

Delving into pregnancy and finding more accurate homeopathic remedy improved the results in the children but the system needed refinement. To me, the most troubling aspect of going through the pregnancy was that the father was essentially cut out of the case-taking process. It felt I was beginning to touch something with a universal quality, but I was still missing a piece of the puzzle. My reasoning was that the father or an adoptive parent should also naturally have equal opportunity as the pregnant mom. I believe the universe is love and love is unprejudiced, by extension, it is only logical that all can access to the information require to heal when well guided.

My search to find a way to take the case through the father and parents of an adopted child marked the beginning of my journey into what I discovered and now call "surrogacy."

CHAPTER 8

Surrogacy

Surrogacy is a concept I characterize as going through the child by an *empathic other.*

Going through the mother's state during pregnancy as a mirror of the child's inner state elicited more in-depth information. But to overcome the presenting challenges of the ASD child and to widen our options, I began to develop a different approach. My goal was to create the possibility, with proper guidance on my part, for the mother and/or father, biological or not, to gain access into the child for the purpose of finding a deeply resonating homeopathic remedy for the child.

To take the case of an ASD child, the speech and language barrier need to be circumvented to access the unspoken inner state. Observing and documenting the child's behaviors does not yield the inner individual experience. As such too much is left to the homeopath's interpretation. Behavior can't be understood beyond stereotypical assumptions, but these same behaviors are the doorways or more explicitly, access into the child when working with a mother or father to get to the core or deepest level. Going through a surrogate is the best and often the only option. The goal is to reach a deeper level, to bring out the experience that reflects most perfectly the state of the child.

At the time, when I was exploring what I came to call "surrogacy" I strongly felt a universal principle at play. My premise was that theoretically anyone can give the case. It shouldn't matter who it is, anyone can reach into the inner state. At the level of what I call "universal mind" we are all connected in the quantum field. "Like everything in the universe, we are connected to a sea of information in a dimension beyond physical space and time. We don't need to be touching or even be near any physical elements in the quantum field to affect or be affected by them, most of the time we are not aware of it because it is not the focus of our attention. The physical body is made of organized patterns of energy and information, which is unified among everything else in the quantum field." (Dr Joe Dispenza) Homeopathic remedies work as a piece of information within this connection at the quantum level through *resonance.*

This principle applies to everyone and probably everything on earth. However, the further away the connection with the child is from the surrogate, the more potentially difficult the process. The idea of the separate self is ego, ego is only an artificial barrier, it is not real.

Parents are the best surrogate candidates because when it comes to their child, these artificial barriers are lowered, most particularly at the time of the child's birth. It is this lowering of the ego that creates the feeling of a deep connection, unconditional love, and empathy. Perhaps it is why the human species has children: To have this experience of connection and unity with another human being. In such a context, when our child feels pain, we experience it. Love is the conductor through which the child's experience of autism can be accessed through a surrogate. Love acts as the conductor when parents vibrate in harmony with their children.

The idea of universal consciousness is nothing new, it has been around for ages. As much as I thought I was spanning uncharted territory of what I called "one mind" and the indivisible divided, the reality is that from ancient Indian texts via Jung to physics and quantum physics, it is a fact except in medicine: We are undivided, we are also one mind and the barriers we perceive are constructs of our minds. In the sphere of case taking the practical application of "One Mind" concept is new, it is a natural step that gives one more opening to give voice to a child who cannot speak to find for him an effective remedy. As stated, it is the challenges autism presents that forced the uncovering of "surrogacy".

So, case taking using surrogacy is the art of lifting artificial barriers between humans to access the expression of illness in an individual. To be successful, the gates of ego must be gently pushed aside. The artificial barriers of what we think is ourselves as individual are willingly and temporarily set aside to access the child's state. Paradoxically, it is a reconnection to the greater whole.

Alice Walker said, "Anything we love can be saved." The perception of oneself must dissolve to reach another. Love removes artificial barriers and parenthood is/can/should be the natural experience of this love without barriers.

Love is the conductor that helps reach the core. Love is the predisposition that creates the connection. Love is emotional understanding of another's experience, which creates the "sensing" of someone else's experience.

To do this, during the initial consultation, the surrogate is guided into the moment, "The only person who exists in the world at this moment is your child." Mom does not exist, Dad does not exist, I don't exist, no one does; only the child. The task at hand is to create complete focus with the individual ego of the surrogate gently guided aside. The best result circumvents the individual's identity of the conscious mind. Removing artificial barriers of separateness allows these unseen channels to open. Understanding the pain of "other" happens here. Automatically sensing someone else's experience, we are diving deep.

Historically the journey into surrogacy happened spontaneously during the initial intake of a particularly eloquent mother. She began to sidetrack and started to speak about her child's difficult behaviors. Normally during an intake, I would gently redirect the mother back to the experience of her pregnancy. This time I felt as if I should not interfere with what she was saying. I clearly had the feeling that something important was happening, I let her continue and realized that she was presenting me with what I now call "doorways" or the paths of least resistance **into** the child. I realized she was having a deeply empathic experience with the behavior she was describing as her child's state. I saw this as a doorway that the right question would open further insights into her child and behind it would be the truth of experience. While she was describing the outward symptom of her child "tapping on everything with his thumb," she was also spontaneously doing it. In essence merging herself with her child. This was the moment I previously described as "strongly feeling a universal principle." Here it was! At this moment there was no need to cut the flow or redirect, but instead listen and allow these doorways to spontaneously open themselves, make note of them and precisely ask the right question to continue deeper into the child. The tapping, the behaviors or habits known as *stims*, are meaningful, the key is finding the meaning behind them through the surrogate.

This is a three-hour process prompted along by carefully worded questions. When the parent has naturally run out of things to say with one question, another is asked to shine a light on other facets of what was previously said. Slowly but surely the answers are more and more refined. It is an effortless process, constantly guided, the parent delves deeper into the unique experience of the child with autism. After countless questions we access the child's central experience. This is when it all comes together, this is where a homeopathic remedy becomes concisely clear. In 2016, I wrote in "One Heart, One Mind" "The first time I was able to reach this deep inside a child on the spectrum (through the mother), I came to realize that I would eventually understand autism from that inside or from the very point of view of the individual on the spectrum". I had no idea then that eight years later the natural development of this process would lead me to write this book, precisely to present the true definition/true center of autism.

Surrogacy allowed access to information that takes us deeper than the conscious mind and therefore deeper into the ailment. Each answer provides an opportunity to reach a deeper in the root of the problem. Ultimately, when we reach deeper levels of analysis each symptom, when taken individually leads to the same inner experience. While incomprehensible at face value, a stim, chronic diarrhea or restlessness, at the depth we reach, combine into one experience. I know we have reached the root of an individual's autism when each symptom evokes the same sensation in the surrogate.

The obvious risk of eliciting the "experience" through surrogacy is that of it being tainted by the surrogate, but that problem resolved itself with experience. It is easy to recognize when the surrogate's rational mind is no longer and the mother, unbeknownst to her, speaks as the child. The process is a dance between questions and answers with the purpose of circumventing the rational and creative brain. When in this state of oneness with a focus on living the child, the child comes through. Universal oneness is non-rational and non-creative. It simply is.

The perception of self on the part of the surrogate dissolves to arrive at a deep remedy for the child. The carefully worded questions create a dance from the left to right brain and vice versa, towards the path of least resistance. Withholding the ego is not an easy task, in fact think it is too much of a leap. I understand that, but the reality of it, is not that much of a leap. There is no need to believe in this but rather to be open to the process and suspend rational thinking for a couple of hours.

The art of surrogate case taking lies in the ability to use questions to produce a dance with the parent between left brain and right brain realms. The process begins with the exploration of various symptoms to elicit descriptive words.

We move back and forth from left brain that rationally names symptoms, "He flaps his hands" to right brain questions, "how does it feel?" that are meant to deepen the understanding, "it feels like there is electricity coursing through the body". As you will see, this back and forth that remains shallow for some time, is only meant to eventually trick the mind to express itself unimpeded by thoughts and feelings. Over time, I came to understand that during a consultation we express ourselves in four different ways:

1. In a rational manner. My child has autism. He has diarrhea 20 times a day, it is always yellow with undigested pieces of food in it. He gets bloated, he flaps his hands and tantrums when we take the iPad away. This is a very rational, factual way of speaking. This is generally the way we begin.

2. Once the facts are exhausted, I might ask a question such as what is the smell of the diarrhea? "It smells sour." It is not uncommon for a diarrhea to smell sour but even *sour* can mean a whole lot of different things. Sour can be that it smells like sour milk, like bread, or yeast. That said, stool is not bread or milk, it is an image and, hence, it is not true. There is no point in taking it into consideration now. If no other information comes out, then I use as a fallback position, we have rubrics "Stool, sour, acid odor, milky" or "Stool, sour, acid odor, like vomit". We have tens of thousands of symptoms repertorized that way. I will explain this in the next chapter, the key is to use these rubrics deeply rather than literally. "When he has diarrhea, does he usually have pain?" "Yes, great pain, he arches his back and cries for a long time." Pain is experiential and spontaneous. As you read this it may sound perfectly logical to you to arch back when in pain but, the child could bend over double or even twist his body. Arching back is potentially very important because movement is spontaneous. It becomes even more important if the child also arches back when someone picks him up and if the same is true when the parent offers food then that symptoms become the language of the body.

3. In the beginning of a consultation, the surrogate veers between facts, story and imagined reasons. Little by little the surrogate's mind runs out of options. There are no more facts or "likes." When this happens the third way of speaking kicks in: Rationalization of feelings or emotionalizing facts.

   Example: The surrogate is asked to describe a particular symptom (behavior or physical symptom) that seems especially vivid or important. Question: "Describe headaches please".

   Response: "I think the pain is sharp". That is a left-brain answer.

Question: "Describe sharp, please".

Response: "It's like being stabbed with a knife". That is creative, it is a right brain answer. It is a comparison, that is truthfully yet not likely, as most people imagine what it is like to be stabbed but have not experienced it. I ask to explain further.

Response: "It is stabbing because (rationalizing) when we massage him, he feels better." Of course, there is no straight-line logic between stabbing and massaging the head. One does not lead to the other but during the consultation this kind of justification happens frequently. The impetus is, unbeknown to the parent, for the mind to remain in control and my goal is to get past the mind.

We expand questions into different areas such as food desires or aversion, obsessive behaviors, dreams, any physical ailment, and, most particularly, acute illness or conditions when life has come to a standstill. All of it is a free flow process, one subject does not automatically come after another, it is all free, unencumbered by predetermined ideas. Little by little, with symptoms such as "diarrhea," "flapping," "fear," or "anxiety" some words repeat. For example, "acidic" could come from different anchor points such as fear and diarrhea. An acidic diarrhea is not uncommon, but for a fear it is. Slowly, uncommon words start to crowd the intake and become the backbone of the code that can translate into a remedy for the child.

4. Simultaneously, the parent answers move to subconscious. The answers become less logical, that is what we want, as in the above example of fear... acidic. I recall a mom talking in this increasingly non-rational, non-creative way, about eating "heavy" and "spicy" pumpkin. As the consultation progressed, the theme of "heavy" and "burning" repeated with several different symptoms. In the mind of a homeopath that is pure gold, the non-sense makes complete sense. That is what is important. The remedy turned out to be *Ferrum Sulphuricum*. Simply explained, symbolically iron is "heavy", and sulphur is "burning". The spontaneity of the answers is not answered by the mind but by the subconscious. To her, "heavy pumpkin" and "burning" didn't lift an eyebrow. The beauty of speaking from subconscious is that it feels perfectly normal, she didn't realize it was not rational and that is exactly what is needed.

To be able to reach in the child in such a manner depends on how much we are willing to suspend our perceived selves and let go of our identity to become someone else. In other words, how much are we willing to adapt to what the situation requires, namely in this case, relieve the suffering of a child. This is not an unknown concept. A politician such as Bill Clinton was well known for having his "thumb on the pulse of the American people". That is one level of synergy. An actor taking on a character in its most detailed feelings and sensations is another. A parent doing this for her child is a natural extension of this process much like a musician getting lost in her music or an athlete going in the zone. The process is well known and applies to countless situation except in the medical realm.

The process is a continual deepening evocation of consciousness and accessing the inner child versus the rational thought. Going from the rational to spontaneous irrationality, with no logical thread connecting point A to point B, has tremendous potential. As the words of the state of the child keep repeating, the sub-conscious is accessed. With experience repeated over and over across different situations invariably leads to great remedies.

When the parent reaches in the zone, the stodginess of belief lifts and is replaced by ease. The words are far more meaningful because they no longer match any rational logical description. The parent is literally living the pain and merging with the Vital Force (VF) of the child. The pure experience of disorder leads directly to the qualities of the remedy and its source. It is a wonderful process and the result after the remedy is given are always brilliant as symptoms such as hyperactivity that seem so engrained in the patients lift off and calmness is restored at times startingly within a few days.

Certainly, given that the process of surrogacy is quite foreign some people are so deeply anchored in themselves it can prevent a complete lifting of the self that seemingly separates us all. Given this represents a significant percentage of parents I had to look further than surrogacy to solve more cases and improve the results

CHAPTER 9

The Homeopathic Analysis Stages

Each case is analyzed according to specific symptomatology most particularly that which is considered "strange, rare and peculiar" (SRP).

For example, when a mother tells me that her daughter is flapping her hands throughout the day, while I understand that is a very difficult symptom to live with, I do not take it into consideration in my analysis because it is not uncommon, nor strange for an individual on the spectrum. However, that symptom, and all the others will be noted to use as reference during subsequent follow-ups to see if they have diminished. The analysis of a case is a three-pronged method that takes into consideration stages and phases. There is little doubt that through understanding autism to its core, the analysis has been automated as the stage for autism is overwhelmingly 12 and a phase will automatically be a 7.

Let us see how and why stages are so important.

ANALYSIS OF THE STAGES:
There are 18 stages. Understanding these stages is a cardinal point of analysis in all homeopathic cases. They represent our modus operandi (M. O.) in life as well as in disease. Each one is characterized by a lack of adaptation within a larger bell curve cycle from beginning to cresting, and

then from losing on to total breakdown. Each point or stage embodies a deeply anchored pattern of action and reaction of a person not only during illness but in life as well. As such, it is interesting to add this knowledge when we interact with people in general. Each stage represents a specific way patients handle illness and most situations in life itself. Stages are also called miasmas. They are the "how" the illness is handled or coped with, according to subconscious perception of the situation. The stage perception characterizes how deep, how chronic, and how acute the illness is experienced. It is not conscious thinking for anyone, it is very much a subconscious process but upon analysis of words chosen to describe illness and suffering there is invariably a set Modus Operandi for each stage that is defined by pace, itself revealing how the disease is perceived. Conjunctly, when we have a "how" there is the "what" of what is felt, perceived, and finally experienced which is embodied by the sensation. The sensation is another aspect of case analysis.

Reversely, the stage is also sensed by the people who are close or take care of the patient daily. As we will see, their reactions are also reflected through common language used that is invariably in tune with the miasmatic block. Most of the language and therapies used in the treatment of autism are set around the modus operandi of stage 12. In my previous book "One Heart, One Mind" I demonstrate through the "surrogacy method" of case taking that both; the how and the what, indeed the modus operandi AND the sensation can be experienced by someone else, most often the mother, I call "The First Witness" but first I'll give a quick overview of how Stage 12 operates.

OVERVIEW OF STAGE 12.
After much experience and observations, as a matter of homeopathic analysis autism is a stage 12 condition. This does not mean that only remedies from stage 12 will be prescribed though it is very unlikely that a child can be reversed fully to neurotypical without one.

As stated, we all operate within a range of action and reaction; all illnesses do, so do children on the spectrum. Stage 12 represents the Modus Operandi (M.O.) of a child on the spectrum. The autism M.O. revolves around the axis of chaos and control. The body, the behaviors, the emotional and the mental state of a child on the spectrum are all in a state of chaos. To alleviate this sense of chaos, the child wants to line things up, keep strict routine, recite the alphabet, count numbers, or repeat phrases heard on TV like a mantra. All these activities, symptoms help make the child feel in control of pains and inner physical sensations within the body and mind. They don't heal the child, in fact the more they are present the worse the child is, but they do however slightly, relieve the sense of chaos experienced by the child. Disrupting or attempting to eliminate that compensation can be severely painful to a child on the spectrum and the consequence is often very violent escalation. A parent might be able to control flapping of hands, but that symptom might quickly be replaced with scratching his face instead. Out of all stages, Stage 12 likes to exert the most control. The reaction to a disruption is often one that can resemble that of a tyrant with external expression of great violence at simply hearing "no" with the result of punching walls or banging the head on the floor. The least important issue can trigger enormous tantrums that can last for days. Stage 12 fights everything because a "Stage 12 person" must have control. Stimming is compensatory behavior to the child on the spectrum and is vital for the child to stay sane no matter how disturbing it is to the people around him. In turn the stimming often drives the parents or therapist to the edge of insanity and their own M.O. is to want to control them by any means. In other words, the reverse application of dictatorial behavior justified by "for his own good" argument is applied.

Stage 12 individuals feel threatened from all directions: Front, back, right, left side, and everywhere in between these points. Under such perceived living conditions all is suspicious and threatening so a great amount of energy is spent to control the environment. That is essentially how most people on the spectrum come to see the world. Children on the spectrum don't like to be videotaped for that reason. "I know I am not behaving normally but I can't do anything about it, what is going to happen to me? "I know I am not behaving properly, don't show me that way." They instinctively dislike being shown, which brings out a deep feeling of inadequacy and not in control of the situation. Order like lining things up or putting an object in a specific place becomes of utmost importance. It makes things look seemingly perfect, but in reality, it is an over perfection.

Perfection is a concept that is itself very misunderstood. Perfection is commonly understood as flawless or faultless but that is not at all what perfection is. By definition, perfection accepts flaws, and in fact even finds beauty in them. What is commonly accepted as perfect, flawless is overdone or exaggerated. Michael Jordan was the best basketball player ever, he was perfect, yet he didn't make all the baskets. Obama came out of nowhere and slid by seemingly without any effort. That is stage 10, ease and perfection precisely because the flawed human aspect is there, he had zero credentials. Stage 12 individual on the other hand over does and overpowers.

Some famous people I suspect operating through stage 12 remedy are for example the Kardashians. Overdoing their lives and making up their faces to a ridiculous point of flawlessness is just that. Skin deep is stupid yet their style has certainly influenced a whole swash of the population.

Donald Trump exaggerations and refusal of anything that is remotely critical are met with extreme reactions also representative of Stage 12. Martha Stewart is another, all is so overly in its place, the garden rows as straight as an arrow, every utensil has its own place, the wreath on the door is exactly the right color. All is so overly controlled nothing is left to chance.

Now let's see Stage 12 in perspective of all the other stages as it will make the arc easier to visualize each Modus Operandi within the whole cycle of the action and reaction, process of construction and destruction.

Stage 1:
The beginning. This is the stage of impulsivity. There is little to no think-ing of what is needed to achieve or consequences of doing anything. It is a very immature M.O., its essence is very simple minded. Action is taken without any reflection; it is an impulse much like an itch must be scratched. All actions are always taken single handedly. There is no time to discuss

any details of projects. There is no shred of doubt even though the person has zero experience in what he is about to enterprise whereas skepticism and study is required when one gets an idea. Stage 1 therefore can be very manic. Bipolar is a consequence of this stage, not surprisingly Lithium, which is commonly prescribed for this illness, is the first element (stage 1), on the left of the second line of the table of elements.

Example: This is the kind of person who at a party interjects himself into a group without being introduced and makes spontaneous comments completely off topic. Eventually everything fails or rather nothing can succeed. Reading this you may think, oh this my little Johnny, interjecting himself inappropriately to talk about dinosaurs. We will see that each stage consecutively builds on the previous one, so stage 12 has an aspect of Stage 1, much like an aspect of Stage 2 etc.... as well.

In illness, we call this stage acute. Actions are taken as if life itself depends on it. It is a reflex action, run! There is danger, the fever is 105F not doing anything is insane. ICU is very much a stage 1 environment. It's life and death. Naturally, in homeopathy we have remedies that specifically cover all stages. In a failed stage 1, panic, terror, and fright ensues. This can look like some autism M.O. but it is not.

Stage 2:
The lonely stage 1 of impulsivity and thoughtlessness behind, stage 2 M. O. is to observe. In a sense this is the true stage 1. They don't want to be seen, they are unsure and shy. They feel judged right away without any reason to justify the feeling and from there easily feel humiliated and hurt. Given that they feel judged just by being looked at they are very sensitive to what others say and easily feel criticized. They don't feel right entering a group. It is very difficult for them to find their place. They underestimate themselves as well so they easily adapt to other's opinions and behaviors. The "yes" man, their shyness makes them look innocent and unharmful, their sense of observation can be prized by others.

Example: They stay right by the door at the party. They feel protected there, they don't engage, it is their security.

In illness, there is an intense crisis that requires a short effort. It is sub-acute, intense effort and all returns to normal. It is like mild food poisoning, by and large nothing serious but we react by going to the emergency room. If one is exposed to contaminated food or water it can lead to typhoid, not life threatening but it needs emergency care, homeopathic or allopathic treatment.

Do notice what is best termed as the speed of these stages. As we go up in stages the speed will diminish and by the time we reach the top of the cycle or bell curve the speed of illness will pick up speed again on the other side. The difference is, in the early stage one is trying to save life but on the other one is trying to avoid death.

Stage 3:
Someone operating out of this stage compares, or scans which is more than observing. Interestingly, one can find the element scandium in the third column. Scan means there is discernment of the observations. They are unsure but they try. Comparing means only that, they don't come to a decision as there is still much doubt. Scanning the options is a good word for this stage. There is a sense of superficiality but there is an active process though it will end in discouragement or non-commitment.

In illness this stage is like ringworm which is characterized by the itch. The itch represents the desire to get to moving. Danger or the perception of it as in the first two stages is much less, this is more anxiety than fear. It is more like a fear of falling rather than fear of starting.

Example: This individual is walking the room, looking, and listening to people talking among each other. She might join a group after scanning the conversations and people, but she is so nervous she excuses herself. It is like parallel play in a child.

Stage 4:
There is enough confidence to establish something. Observations and comparisons are done, they feel they know something and can have a go at it. They feel empowered, the ridicule is not there at first, but once reality

hits they feel very unsure and get panicky. Panic or nervous breakdown is a result of having engaged, the stakes are higher but they can still back out. Sort of the same feeling when a child's feet can no longer touch the bottom of the pool. There is venture but they don't go any further. My daughter, Florencia and I were relaxing at a lakeside in France when a group of divers showed up. As we were looking at them get themselves ready with all their gear, I noticed what turned out to be a first timer, an adult and although he was in three feet of water, he was so anxious he was literally shaking like a leaf. As he was contemplating going under for the first time, he backed out. That is stage 4. He has committed to doing something, but the commitment is very fragile.

In illness, this is the age of measles or mumps. The average age of these two is between 6 and 15 years old. This is the age range when children venture out of the protection of the parents but quickly return. It's the time of the first bike. It is important to note that while both illnesses claimed deaths in the past the prevalence of medical access today makes them very benign. Vaccination policies were put in place during the confluence of great scientific push and massive amounts of people moving to cities. Working out of the house, the parents could not nurse the kids who went to very schools. On the other hands, the countryside was totally deprived of doctors, vaccination made sense. Unfortunately, the natural process of these illnesses is not seen as part of a fortifying process for the body and immune system. Not getting sick is still seen as a good thing yet today, most people have instant access to health care that can very easily treat measles or mumps. From the homeopathic point of view there are enough homeopathic remedies that have shown to be extremely effective over many decades against these illnesses to dramatically minimize the risks.

Perhaps it is why the first generation to be fully vaccinated, The Millennials, the first generation of kids to not have the physical experience of overcoming minor illnesses, is the first generation to have difficulties establishing themselves in the world remaining indecisive about their role in society and not officially moving out of the house. It is interesting that Stage 4 keywords are door, gate, bridge, key, ratify.

Example: She knows the people at the party, she carefully announces she is getting engaged. Or it is someone engaging properly in a group at the party with proper repartee, but the conversation becomes too deep, he become nervous and leaves. While Stage 3 discovers, Stage 4 is amazed. Wow, but the feeling won't last because life is bound to get more complicated. This is often referred to as beginner's luck. This is not stage 1 which announces irreverent of anyone or anything. Signing a lease for example, getting your own keys is Stage 4. Another example of Stage 4 is when you give the keys of your apartment to the person you love.

Stage 5:

The announcement has been made and now the need is to prepare for the next step. The tasks are very big, too big. It is easy to get discouraged or disappointed during the planning phase. That is very much Stage 5. There are so many options to weed through they can't make up their mind, postponement is the best option. Making the announcement had seemed so easy. Now they cry every day because "this is so hard". It is also the stage of the first prototype. It is easy to think it won't work. The prototype has flown which is a step further from stage 4 but still giving up will limit the loses. It is also the stage of bulimia. I eat but once I ate, I have to vomit because I am going to gain weight. I had a case in my early years of practicing of a dancer who was taking classes six days a week. Acting and dance schools in New York are full of such students. They are always preparing for auditions they seldom go to. They are constantly preparing for something they want but remains ethereal.

Example: In our hypothetical person at a party. She is joining groups but there are so many. So many conversations. I wish everything were simpler. There is so much choice, I don't know. I should not have said so much. I expected too much out of this party, it is a disappointment. I need to scale back, sit down and chill.

STAGE 6:

The proof is in the pudding. The wavering of stage 5 is gone, now "I will prove that I am capable". This is the stage of accepting the challenge, there is no turning back. These people look for or always perceive a challenge.

They love it, the feeling of hesitation is behind them, they can grab the bull by the horns and harness the situation. Running away is no longer an option as it was in stage 2 through 5. Turning around is not an option, it's a go. There certainly is risk involved but "someone's got to do it, why not me?" is Stage 6 state of mind. They control their fear, this is a very public stage of courage and bravery. They want the feat to be seen in order to be proved correct. When I was eight years old, my teacher made a comment about books and within that conversation I said that my parents own the smallest book on earth. I explained that it must be very carefully handled with tweezers and that each pages contained the same prayer written in many different languages. My teacher promptly dismissed me. The next day, I came back with it, proudly and mockingly showed the prized possession to my teacher in front of the other pupils. I had to prove my word, produce the object, and didn't shrink from doing so.

Example: At the party, he has to prove he fits in and show everyone that he can hold his own within the group. It is the stage of hazing in school. I can take some abuse to belong.

STAGE 7:
Now that the basics have ascertained one quickly finds out that he needs to learn more. The subject that one proved he could do needs to be studied further to perfect it. This is the stage of learning techniques, facts, getting feedback and going back to the drawing board. The doubts are no longer whether the chosen road is correct but rather how to approach and walk the path in the most efficient way. These people can get stuck in the technical parts of the project. Jeff Van Gundi was a coach for the NY Knicks basketball team. He was recognized for knowing all sorts of facts and details about his opponents. He overwhelmed his players with some much technical data they could not win. Not so incidentally you'll find the element Technetium in the seventh column of the table of elements. Van Gundy knew so much he should have won but he got so mired in the facts and complexities, the game became too technical to win. Another example of this stage can be found during the war in Afghanistan. In 2010, the U.S. commanding officers requested a chart of Afghanistan tribal complexities. What came back was a PowerPoint slide so densely packed of facts that

General McChrystal remarked "The day we understand that slide, we'll have won the war". It is too much information, so much so that the central point gets lost. Following this presentation, General James Mattis said, "PowerPoint makes us stupid". Jeff Van Gundy retired from coaching and became a basketball commentator on TV, a profession that is well suited for pouring out statistics to fill the air.

Example: At the party, our imaginary friend knows the names, likes and dislikes of everyone but those facts while useful for individual acts of kindness don't contribute to the fun of the party. This stage (as others) might make you think of Asperger's kids who join in awkwardly with facts and details about dinosaurs or whatever other subject they happen to be interested in. That is true, but it also points out to stage 1 as well, the introduction is often sudden and unasked for. Keep in mind again, that each stage builds on the previous one. A stage 7 individual has within himself all the other stages as well, 1 through 6.

Stage 8:
The path is certain, the books have been studied, the pressure is mounting, time is running out. There is no thought of postponement as in stage 5. This is the stage of the hard push, get in the final four. The work is massive, the study is for the final. Opposition is not welcome at all; this is the stage where it felt the most. One is bracing for the worst but there is inner strength. Perseverance is the keyword. It is the stage of overcoming; calculations are still taking place but only to pump oneself up that all is good. "I don't have to know this, concentrate, persevere and succeed can be mine" which is within reach now. There is no distraction, only focus, no time for celebration but it can be imagined. It is the "I Have a Dream" speech, the struggle and opposition are organized. It is Sisyphus rolling the rock up hill, or in the movie "The Mission" when Robert de Niro is climbing the waterfall with all his possessions. Stage 8 can also be perceived as doing penance, one must push through. A different facet of it is the marathon runner who falls apart at the finish line because it is so hard. De Niro, as Rodrigo in the film "The Mission" is released of his load by an Indian and suddenly cries uncontrollably. Success can be attained but will be experienced and remembered that way, as a very difficult struggle.

Example: Our friend has been accepted, he has studied the individuals and has made friends within the group, now he has to do things for the group that are of questionable nature.

Stage 9:

The final push, almost at the top, success is within reach, it can be actualized. Nearly all the work has been done, the right decisions, the right compromises made. The dress rehearsals are in the final stage. Capacity has built, success is on the verge of becoming reality but there is a blunder. It is when people say, I could smell it, I could touch it. While stage 8 is the true mountaineer forcing himself through, stage 9 fails 20 meters from the top. Stage 9 people are confident, they win but there is the remnant of fear of something unforeseen when all will be lost. So much has been done, nearly all has been done, in fact this stage should be easy, but they call it off. I am not going. Somehow this option out is better than going the last step and not making it. This is the eternal second. Scotty Pippen playing second fiddle to Michael Jordan. In France, we had Poulidor, a cyclist who came in second three times and five times third, in The Tour de France. He was known as "the eternal second" though he made podium more times than anyone else.

Example: Our friend is the maid of honor, she has been instrumental in organizing and be a support for her best friend's wedding, she has written her speech all is ready but on the morning of she decides she won't do it.

Stage 10:

The goal is reached. One is at the top. This is a natural top, like Obama who becomes editor of "Harvard Journal" seemingly without any effort. Then he becomes Senator and then President naturally bypassing much more experienced candidates. The confidence is very natural, it is doubtless. All these previous stages are internalized within their Modus Operandi. It is Cinderella. She shows up and she is the star. One downfall is haughtiness on the part of these people. Michael Jordan made trash talk a household word. Obama thought his views and thoughts were so evidently better, more intelligent that everyone should follow him, but politics is not about getting to the top, it is dealing with everyone else who is not.

Example: Our imaginary guy walks in a room and simply commands it, people are happy to be considered by and are attracted to this person who seems to have a certain glow. Most commonly stage 10 people are physically quite present, very suave people. You can't miss them, they attract others. Righteousness is one unwanted quality of Stage 10 people. They can see their status so obvious that others should be able to do the same. This is Michael Bloomberg who tells Senator Elizabeth Warren she too could have been a billionaire. One drawback of this stage can be experienced as a precarious situation requiring fixes and rigid ideas all the time. "It's a lonely place at the top" is a good saying for Stage 10.

Stage 11:
While stage 10 naturally belongs, succeeds etc. according to what is at hand, stage 11 having past the summit, feels he needs to maintain his position. Preserving or conserve. The tomatoes are ripe, they will be conserved to lengthen the amount of time they can be eaten. While the purpose of the ascent is to get to the top, the perception starting with stage 11 is to preserve or protect what has been gained. One can get busy extending the win. This is like the movie "My Greek Wedding" that becomes a Broadway show, a book, a TV show etc. They enjoy the fruits of the success and expend on it. There is a certain stiffness that comes with it too, the sequel is never quite the same. One understands instinctively that getting to the top is not the end. Stage 11 individuals want to extend the winnings, he is constantly recounting his exploits, not for himself though that keeps him plugged in to the success but also to share it and people come to be inspired. They share it with others, there is a certain benevolence. Senator john Mc Cain was very much a stage 11 person. He never saw a war he didn't like, in the sense of a noble cause, he wanted to spread the good things America had to offer. His sense of stage 11 allowed him to expand himself through torture in Vietnam and his story was always used as an inspiration for others. Stage 11 achieves very well but is not commonly your straight A student, instead he has natural affluence or privilege. It is the stage when the mountaineer has just left the summit, still reeling from his success he knows the slope is slippery and one need to maintain vigilance. He knows more people die going down that going up. The other side was the birth and the different

dangers on the way to blooming; starting with state 11, the general goal is to prevent death.

Example: Stage 11 people come to the party and liven it up. They are well received; they have a rich disposition, they know their worth, no need to flash it. They know what they need to do and make everyone feel very privileged in their sharing and protection.

Stage 12:
This is the most important and primary stage of an individual on the spectrum. All the stages integrate the stage prior as an evolutionary process. Each stage does not happen in a vacuum but includes the behaviors of all the stages that come before it. The behaviors and experiences of stage 12 include therefore all the behaviors of Stage 1 through 11 plus 12.

Stage 12 is the stage of fighting, overdoing and exerting power. As we have crossed on the other side of the bell curve, starting with Stage 11, one feels the grip on success is getting looser. Losing begins to feel real but it is not an option. Lose once, lose always, fight is the only option or chaos will ensue. This person feels the slippery slope under his feet, and it feels like oblivion. It is not stage 16 that is deeply broken as we will see, the point here is that control is slipping. At stage 10 all is under control, in fact things just fall in place. To have a sense of control here one must fight. The fear of decline is enormous so he must exercise optimal control for it to not show. Suspicion is quite great though not so much in children but going into corners, under the table or blanket is a soft representation of that feeling, eventually, if a homeopathic remedy is not given "real suspicion" develops. Suspiciousness in ASD kids is represented in the deep dislike to be on video. Showing a less than desirable image is not an option at times, even when deep on the spectrum, with grave conceptual inability there is what seems to be an instinctual quality to prevent showing weakness. Anything short of total freedom is experienced as opposition. In that sense, with forceful behavior such as throwing themselves on the floor, screaming etc. children surpass the ability of most parents to control their kid. They endure the ABA, the therapies, the doctors and the many discussions in front of them. Eventually they feel they are a disappointment and lash out on the therapist that pushes them far above their abilities. Contextually they know they can't talk and join in. They are not becoming what is expected as Stage 12 itself is perceived as needing to put in a superhuman effort. Level two patients fight to overcome their autism, it is felt as a superhuman effort. Most of the time they are aware or have a sense of what is said, they sense there is something wrong with them and all the repetitions affirm the shortcoming. Stage 12 has an image issue in the sense that they are over doing to prevent loss.

The prefix for this stage is Re. Repeat is very much what ABA is based upon, it is also what individual on the spectrum do as well. Repeating gives them a sense of control, having to repeat feels like a loss of control. Repeat until the repetition is automatic. This is awful in many ways. I recall a patient who was "taught" to say she was hungry. This seemed of primary importance to parents as she never asked for either food or water. One day she said "hungry". The parents were so happy, gave her the food she seemed to like. Filled with excitement, they waited to see her eat but she didn't. She didn't know what she was saying, she was just repeating.

This is the stage where the opportunity is given to REthink our lives. It can mark the moment of REdemption or REverse and change his ways but in sickness one can't do that. "And the day came when the risk to remain tight in a bud was more painful than the risk it took to blossom" - Anais Nin. 1

Stage 8 requires perseverance through the final push but the M.O. of stage 12 is to not RElinquish hence the perseverance behaviors. Stage 8 is often by himself or a small group to get to the top but as Stage 12 personality is sub-consciously losing grip, he looks for prompts from others, reads the atmosphere in his need to fight. He is very adept at recruiting or involving a lot of people or systems in his life.

The community speaks of reversing autism. These terms are not accidental, they come from the sub-conscious of the community that serves this illness as it is steeped deeply into it. They spontaneously come to the community that understands that world of specific illness and its needs.

Certainly, there is much suspicion in the parents of children on the spectrum. Suspicion regarding vaccines and the alienation that ensues. Suspicious of foods and Big Pharma. The FDA is not trusted at all by the community. It is also the suspiciousness towards yeast, microbes, parasites, heavy metal, this is why parents are so convinced of them as the culprits.

Example: This individual arrives at our party and quickly makes grand claims that the world has so many problems, we are losing everything, prevent complete loss, only he can reclaim the torch. "Make America great again" is a perfect Stage 12 slogan, no wonder Trump's message resonated deeply in the community.

All these stages show us how we all act and react to a stressor or illness according to our perception. As such, it important to recognize the M.O. of a child as a crucial understanding to be able to parent accordingly. Certainly, a Stage 2 child should be parented very differently from a Stage 12 child. The most effective method of parenting will be the one that matches the child temperament the most accurately. It is commonly said that there are as many parenting methods as there are parents. The cliché is rather poor and certainly non-descript, for one, shouldn't there be as many methods as there are children? My observations tell me that in real life, there are essentially two parenting methods.

Here is an adapted version of an article I wrote with my 10-year-old daughter Florencia.

Simply stated, the first might be called the laissez-faire method. It is the best friend, child king or queen elevated on a pedestal that leads to aggrandizing ego of the little Einstein. Mesmerized by their progeny, the parents ask the child to solve situations, make premature decisions or give an opinion beyond her years of maturity. When there is a problem, such as crying or more likely a temper tantrum the method to stop it is rationalization. A totally inappropriate in the moment as the child cannot process rational adult talk no matter how childishly it is expressed. Curiously parents who adhere to this method revert to rational baby talk when there is a problem. You can hear them at the playground all-the-time. Later, in life as adult, these kids have difficulty making decision on groundless egos. It is part of the "you are smart" problem. Yes, telling most children except the Stage 2 and 3 children, even then in limited dose, "You are smart" is a very bad idea. The problem results after the child has been told so many times that he is smart that when he fails, he has nothing to hang onto. Since failure is inevitable the child will think that he has been lied to, that in fact he is not smart, he knew that all along. This is classic in kids with ADD. So many relationships, self-confidence and egos have been destroyed that way albeit with good intentions that it is keeping a lot of therapists busy.

Perhaps a book should be written on the subject, "Parenting Homeopathically" or "Resonant Parenting". By and large, the friendly method is disliked by the overwhelmingly popular second method, the other side of the same coin, that can best be described as heavy on parental control of children behavior (which despite the bravado is in the end driven by fear).

When the children don't do what they are demanded to do, punishment is applied with "time outs" most often preceded by confrontation, yelling or worse verbal and often physical abuse. Florencia says, "the screaming scares and diminishes the child. The parents scream but when the child begins to do the same the parents don't like it and it becomes a hypocritical situation". One could hardly hear a finer example of a stage 12 kid. This is an extremely powerfully clear statement. Times outs might bring some minimal results for Stage 6 to 8 children but overall, for the purpose of this book, time outs for Stage 12 children are singularly ineffective. Not only can little be built on this, but it is also deeply suppressive and counterproductive, besides being stressful for all involved parents, children, and family. Such violence is exercised to bring about various degrees of submission, effectively robbing the child of his sensitivity, creativity, expressionality and a complete disregard of his emotional needs.

In the end, distilling either method leads to the inevitable conclusion that both methods rest on fear. The first spurs from a need to be best friend with the child, perhaps because the parents were raised in a disciplinarian environment. As a parent the need to connect on friendly terms to avert past childhood experiences inevitably becomes the weakness that is taken advantage of by the child, not from malicious intent but rather because it is a button, that can be pressed. The second is based on such fear of not having the child "turn" a certain way, or from a strong need to get "respect". Oppressive parenting, most often by a repressive hand is needed to mold the kid to teach her about "the real world". The impediment to freedom leads to the de facto teenage crisis. What is amazing about this is that we don't even pause for a second to ask ourselves, as parents why is there a teen crisis? There is never a pause, in this all-knowing parental model that there could be something wrong, that teen crisis itself is perhaps due to our parenting. A need to forcefully break away from the oppressive hand. With this model sympathy and giving are regarded as weaknesses. Is there any wonder the child wants to leave?

Flo sees one problem with discipline as an observation of adults saying to do one thing but themselves not doing what they say. Do as I say not as I do situation. An easy example might be tolerating the child on the phone, opportunistically to be able to watch TV in peace. Once the football game over, the parent asks the child to get away from the phone, at which point it is difficult for the child to give it up. Make no mistake about it, the child is aware of opportunism displayed and now feels that it is his time to be opportunistic, yet such a situation often devolves into the demands getting stronger ending up in argument. In day-to-day life, this is what most parent practice. Such a situation can be diffused before it even starts simply by communicating that you will watch the game and that after that, you would like to do A, B, C or D or ask what your child wants right after the game.

There is a third way, the plus one, I call auxiliary. It is a combination of the two, a potpourri of tolerance, discipline which at face value may sound good but in reality, leads to a cacophony or incongruent parental decisions often spurred by immediate demands.

It is from this bird's eye view that I decided I was going to do neither. Where neither my child nor I would experience fear, neither would experience being taken advantage of, or neither of us would feel impeded by the other. That should lead to the feeling of being completely open and accepted, in turn leading to free speech. That, in family dynamics is called belonging. In belonging there is safety, respect, rest, and love. That is the most solid base possible. This is the only way to build a relationship, in fact under the maintenance of these conditions it builds itself. Thankfully as a homeopath I am deeply versed in resonance so instinctively, as a parent it was my responsibility to create the conditions to be in perpetual resonance with my child and vice versa, for Florencia to be in resonance with me. I don't see how there is another way to develop a deeply understanding, meaningful and loving relationship. Understanding of an individual, cannot happen in his opposition nor in opportunity nor in keeping up a façade.

To that end, I turned the whole parent child relationship on its head. I started to view, as a matter of exercise, the relationship from my child's point of view. "If I were in her shoes?" was my question, after all compassion is the ability of seeing the other person's point of view.

Parental advice from my listening tour of Florencia
I understand that the following strays from parenting a child on the spectrum, but if there is one child in the family on the spectrum there is a good chance that another child while not on the spectrum can be of stage 12 M.O.

Children must listen to us because we know better. I cannot think of a worst statement than this. It is in essence dismissive, diminishing, insulting and disrespectful. I know it is a difficult exercise, but once you put this notion aside and actually listen to the child all the time, not occasionally, but literally all the time, you would be amazed at how often children are correct in their feelings and perception of a given situation as well as eloquent at expressing their feelings. Florencia says she sees parents "take advantage of their kids by blaming them for their behaviors". Logic would have it that the top-down parent, if so in charge and responsible should be the one who should be blamed. If there is failure, then by that logic set by the (all knowing) parent is wrong. Florencia is correct in her statement;

blaming is taking advantage of the child. As soon as that happen the relationship is on rocking ground. Nothing peaceful can come out of that. In the long term, either taking or being taken advantage of will result later in life because that is what was learned.

You might think that my relationship with Florencia is flawless, but I beg to differ. While I make it my responsibility to always listen and teach, listening it is not as easy as it seems. For example, I often tell Flo that "all will be fine" "not a big deal" when she expresses deep concerns. Nothing wrong in saying "all will be fine" right? Well, one day she told me "Dad, you always think everything will be fine" and at that moment I realized that saying what I thought were words of comfort was dismissive of her concerns. I immediately apologized to her, I felt badly and expressed my feelings. This taught me one thing. Even with years of taking responsibility for fostering a non-argumentative relationship that has led to a mutually respectful deeply loving relationship, a never-ending endeavor to make it better my relationship with my daughter should never be on automatic. The key is parental versatility.

It may be becoming clear now that most of the yelling and thereby the punishment is not necessary and in fact probably is counterproductive. I understand parents, are often at their wits end, feeling they have "tried everything" that no yelling may sound too good to be true. The only way to get Little Johnny off the tablet is to literally snatch it away from him.

As with everything, it should all start with being conscious of our parenting philosophy to be able to not only change our course but the course of our children's lives. The disclaimer here, is that a reversal of behaviors does not happen overnight but with applied focus, your change of behavior will begin to bear fruits after several challenging months. There is a rather simple reason for that. Arguments follow a precise pattern each time. All relationships follow well-worn emotional actions and reactions patterns that are integral to our perception of the world at large.

So, which within these two categories do we fall or lean into? How do we get to the point where we can enjoy our children rather than view them as chores or drag on our lives? Are we destined to struggle for years with the hope that at some point there will be a miraculous turn around? How can we expect years of hurt to magically disappear? Can we really expect that somehow this one parent -child venerated relationship will be different? Why should it be? This implies a lot of wishful thinking. There is nothing holy about a child parent relationship. Estrangement is far more common than we think and most often begins in childhood.

Indeed, the following African proverb tells this story very well.

"Peace in your house will be a counterpoint to the enmity in the world".

No matter the situation, there is an opening for synergy, true resonance between parent and child. It is possible, the first and most important key is to begin of being aware of antagonism and fears. It is our foremost responsibility, the sooner one starts the better. The first step is actually very simple and effortless. The first thing, one should do is visualize a two-way street with you and your child on it. The distance between the two of you reflects your current situation so be honest, don't manipulate what spontaneously shows in your mind's eye. Every day, you take the responsibility to bring the two of you together. There is a long term as well as hindsight visualization. There is also a short term one to reflect near present and future. Every day you work so that this visualization becomes more and more even as well as closer and closer. The key to making this happen can be summed up in one word. Versatility.

A successful parenting career is a multi-dimensional and a highly creative process. Creativity is essential to not only avoid the pitfalls of the emotional ruts mentioned earlier but critical to keep growing which entails the number one ability to have: constant adjustments. I literally cherish every minute with Florencia, I like to say we have a father daughter relationship of course, but I am also the uncle, the clown, the teacher, the bad neighbor, we are great friends. I am unconditionally nurturing, yet I can be deeply fatherly as well, my radar is fixed on having resonance with each other to create ease and freedom for the both of us. Different moments require a different hat. For example, let's say we are reviewing math on Khan academy. A chore kind of thing for most people. At first sight, you might label that teacher role but 7th grade math is well behind me so I may turn her into the teacher to teach me when I see she is at ease. That give confidence. I may play clown and fake not knowing so she can deepen her understanding while having fun. Then I might become competitive and challenge her into doing a few equations. Agility is required, to make it easy for the both of us. In the end, she generally wants to do more and now when I say we are doing Khan on Saturday, her answer is "OK". One may feel like this is bending too much to the need of the child, but I beg to differ. Stay true to yourself and be it known that by being versatile you are teaching it as well. Versatility is key to success in business as well as most endeavors. The extraordinary relationship I have with Flo grew out of versatility and visualizing the two-way street.

Sonny comes in from school with that fatigued gait that makes him drop on his bed as if he had just climbed Mount Everest (twice for good measure) and every day he drops his backpack in the middle of the living room. Every day you complain. "Pick up your bag" once in a blue moon it "works" after repeating several. Sometimes you don't bother and other days you blow a gasket. The potpourri, auxiliary method. What is your attitude going to be starting today that will start to develop respect, consistency, understanding and love? Which hat are you going to invent to make dropping the bag in his bedroom. It is the hat that will have resonance with your child at that moment. It may be that you will explain how disrespected you feel. You will say that by covering him with kisses, right? If your husband wakes up every morning and tells you, you look great every morning you won't believe him, right? But because of consistency after some time, you will. Be consistent in finding love that is in your child. People like to say that kids don't come with an instruction manual, that is not true. They are the manual, most of us need to read it. If you complain about your child, your method is not working and therefore needs to be changed, there is no need to defend a method that does not result in a perfect relationship. This is what I seek, because among the many purposes of my relationship with Florencia, to me parenting is part of a larger purpose of building a better society. If we hit children or yell at them that is what the product will do. That is unacceptable.

Historically, the top-down method of parenting reflected factory work conditions, do as I say and don't ask questions. Yet, by watching and reading biographies of creative people who "made it" in life, it seems that they often relate to having very free childhood and deep relationships with, at least one parent. So, if I wanted my child to be "great" and free then that is the model I should follow. This is pure logic to me.

Today's kids are exposed to hundreds of desires a day. Parents feel they have to say "no" all the time. Guess what, you are correct, you are saying no hundreds of times a day. Advertisement is plastered everywhere with one goal in mind to creates desire in a kid's mind and ideally convince the adult that it is good. That is what happened with phone and tablets which today is one of the biggest sources of conflict in families. We are constantly triggered. The reality is while you say "no" a hundred time a day we do say "yes" often out of exhaustion. That one time the child wins negates all the nos. You see, I grew up without any choice whatsoever. I was in the mountains, there were no stores. My playground was going in the mountain or do summersault in hay barns. That was it. No choice and boredom. Two things I wish kids had today.

Solution:

Sit down instead of stop jumping. Positive language. Once we are told to not do something, we do it. Even worst, then we get physical. Stage 12 children love to negotiate. This is also a good skill to have in life.

Solution

There is no one way of doing, for example, use positive language. It is like diet, if we do one thing that one thing won't work in all situations.

Give the child control.

Communicate your feeling, communicate your weaknesses, there is no point in hiding them, your child figured them out a long time ago. For example, Flo knows I am not the most patient person in the world. When she presents me with a situation where I must be patient, I let her know that I am really stretching myself, I describe my experience. Since we have set a two-way street, she becomes aware of it, she helps or even comfort me in a such situation. As parents we are responsible for setting up the two-way street and place our children on it to gradually take on responsibilities.

Solution

Break down your question into bite size question. How was your day in school? is not constructive. Break it down into "I saw a poster on the wall at school about recycling. It looked interesting, do you know what it says?"

Solution

Ask silly questions too. I wonder why the desks are always brown. I wonder if desks with flowers would be better, what do you think? There are a million questions one can ask instead of "How was your day?"

SPECIFIC UNDERSTANDING OF STAGE 12 IN AUTISM CASES.

We have seen how individuals operating out of Stage 12 need to control all elements within their environment with dictatorial behaviors to prevent the feeling of chaos in their lives. They fight for order. Fight does not give much leeway. It is black or white, either you are with me or against me. In their eyes it is a win or lose situation. There is no gray area with this comportment. This is what we see with autism. An absolute need to precisely line up pencils or toys is a Stage 12 quality to prevent chaos. The feeling of loss or rather not wanting to lose explains so much of the autism behaviors. It explains "the logic" of pooping in the diaper rather than the toilet. This feeling is crucial to understand as it is an integral part of the condition. Preventing loss or holding is taken to the extreme, days without going to the bathroom which causes great pains to pass stool that is getting harder, drier, and more difficult to physically get rid of or pass. Even then, once passed with great difficulty it is best to "hold" in the diaper. Likewise, we often hear parents say that "he hates the flushing sound". Yes, that is correct but not the sound itself but rather the effect of the flush is that it will be gone forever. It is not as much sound sensitivity as it is what water does. Water is the bad guy that takes my poop away. Conjunctly, I have noticed the severity of the constipation is often related with the desire to hold one or more toys in the hands and the inability of letting go of it.

STAGE 13

After the stage of fight comes the stage of withdrawal. The position cannot be held. This is a position that is removed from the top. This position is shrunk from what it could have been. One is holding on to obsolete tools, weapons, or manners. There is a sense of being outdated. Those pants looked good at one time, now they are used. This is the moment of lifetime award; the master withdrew a while ago. The spotlight is no longer, it is a kind of coming out of the woodwork. There is an element of mold to this stage. It's like the zucchini that's been too long in the fridge, you cut off the molded piece and use the rest of it.

Physically this represents mycosis or fungal infections such as clearing of the skin in spots. Recurring vaginal infections is stage 13. A lot of biomed physicians talk of candida overgrowth. That is the stage of anti-fungal medications. Very commonly people with such infections stay home. They don't want to be seen in public. How can I go out looking like this? They are very self-convinced of their situation and will argue with others about it. Stage two feels observed, stage 13 is different, they are not weak like Stage 2 they just think that their way was better. It is nostalgia, like leaving a dance, because it is hip hop rather than disco. There is an old-fashioned quality. This is the main reason why going after mold and yeast for kids on the spectrum can only bring marginal benefits. The therapy is not accurate, it is theoretical, it is a checked box in the long list of culprits' integrative medicine blame for illness.

STAGE 14

There is no more power, only formal. This is the stage of the disposed dictator. There is only a mask. There are only remnants of power. It is like the Royal family in England. The only power they have is of a formal facade. You sit down after the queen does. The queen wears a blue brooch to express her like of Europe, she can't prevent Brexit. Her guards are like little lead soldiers. Not surprisingly you will find the element lead in this column. They are distant, their strength lays in the diversion of people or issues. They don't touch the important matters; the pressure is off; they can only rest on their laurels. There are only formalities left, protocols and rules, signing the closing papers. There is stiffness. One of the most well-known British maxims is 'Stiff upper lip". In a more active manner, this is also the stage of the diplomat who does not show his chips. This is the stage of being dis-tracted or dismissed. Distant, discredited, disinterested. This is often the stage when ADD is diagnosed. At first the kiddo was "very smart", his distraction disrupted the class, now he is being dismissed, he will be displaced to the front of the class next to the teacher.

Physically there is a lot of atrophy, this is the stage of Parkinson's with the facial mask. No more expression. Polio is part of this stage.

STAGE 15

This stage marks the beginning of always feeling defeated, of always being on the wrong end of the stick. There always something missing. Within this Stage, one can find Phosphorus, a remedy who profoundly dislike being alone. They feel deeply sympathetic, have a long list of friends they talk to until late at night. They are very appreciated for instinctively know-ing the pain of loss, that is what their M. O. revolves around. This is stage 15 combined with the third series of sociability. Loss of people.

The remedy Arsenicum relates to the fourth series that represents work hence these are people who often lose their job. To compensate for it they are very fastidious, keeping things in order, constantly under the fear of losing. Losing job means going bankrupt. More than bankruptcy, stage 15 is also the stage of surrender or sacrifice. While Stage 12 would never even contemplate such option Stage 15 does and lives it as a motto. This is the firefighter going in the fire to save someone.

STAGE 16

After loss, there are only remnants, the leftovers. The story of Cinderella but without a prince to save her. For example, I gave the remedy Mezereum to a patient with loss of hair and fears of auto-immune diseases, most particularly of having diabetes later in life. I asked her "How do you picture or imagine living with this illness?" "The condition is spreading. It is all dark gray, charcoal color. It is constant suffering without a break, I am completely alone. I am surrounded by ashes, as if there had been a big fire. Not a single color, nothing is growing. I am in a place where all is destroyed, there are no plants, nothing is green. I am sitting on my heels. Everything is gone has been taken. All forms of life are gone. No plant, no animal, or humans. It is survival. How am I going to survive? There is nothing to eat, there is nothing."

This is how she experienced her illness, not necessarily how she lived. I asked a lot of follow up questions, I thought someone was going to pop out of oblivion and make the situation easier, the human race continues but nope! This was her view. Totally stage 16, all is gone. Result after one month: Hair is not falling anymore; the blood numbers are all good. Three months hence: Hair has regrown.

This case also tells a lot about honesty and being real when describing illness or the feeling of it. She could have thrown in a feel-good sentence but that would have thrown the case in a different direction, so I used the rubric: "Delusion, everything is dead". We use the word "delusion" in the sense of feeling and the remedy completely healed her problems.

STAGE 17

"This is the end" as Jim Morrison of The Doors sang so poignantly. Eradication, you're done. Death row, total outcast. All is gone, all has been given up. There is no bond, there is memory. The ship is sinking, it is not despair, it is hopeless despair. In a sense one can feel totally liberated. When the feeling is that all is gone, then there can be no scruple about stealing. When people say "You create your own reality" well, there is truth to it. Our modus operandi whichever one we operate out of is central to that idea. All is final for stage 17, death is here, at any time. Terrorists operate out of this stage. They have written their will; life will end soon. They have spoken as having been liberated when given the oath but the path to that stage is so severely painful, the only way is to let go. Terminal disease. Death is here, they are exiting.

Or they are always an outsider. This is an adult who never felt loved, though could have been loved but never felt it. They might have been banned because their ego is too strong. Whatever the conversation these are the type who somehow bring everything back to themselves. Borderline Personality disorder has that stage 17 behavior. Not having a family might also trigger a stage 17 M.O. Nobody to lose type of feeling. This is why, the life story of criminals is so always very much the same. We may think it is the situation that triggers the M.O. but not necessarily, the willpower to get away from it might be too great to overcome.

One could be banned from a job. It is the stage of being banned for their idea or behavior. Comedians are in the crosshair nowadays. Comedy is a very stage 17 activity. One cannot be scared to bring out what is dissonant within what is "normal" or taken for granted. The lack of fear is there because comedians carry within themselves all the other stages, they see all points of view. This is what makes the humorist understand the ridicule. It is the ridicule of a serious situation that creates change. Stage 2 is the fool who used to accompany kings, he observes and tells the king his observations. He is non-threatening. Stage 17 is Voltaire, who tells the truth criticizing by wits, he is dangerous, he was exiled. It is also Henry Mc Henry character played by Adam Driver in the movie Annette. Stage 17 is the end, there will be a new beginning with Stage 1 after the period of rest of stage 18. It is the convict who has served his sentence and starts his life all over again or the divorced who starts his life again.

Interestingly it is also the stage of climax. A lot of criminals talk about doing the crime as a culmination. Climax is the end. Soon there will be Stage 1 but between the end and new beginning there is a stage of transition.

STAGE 18

It is a stage of transition between the end of all stages or cycles and the beginning of another. It is a stage of rest or meditation. This is the stage where some people find "answers" during meditation. In that case it is a temporary opening rather than a permanent one. One withdraws alone, safe from all that the stages described.

It is the stage of hibernation or cloister or holiday or out of existence. Withdrawn might make us think of autism but autism is not a stage of dormancy as many used to think. Autistic individual fight for comfort within a limited life. Stage 18 does not fight for anything. This is a cocoon stage; the bear is sleeping, another way to look it is, the sperm is swimming. It is a transitional stage from a relationship, or from work, transition from a career to another or transition from a set of ideas to a different set. During those moments one reflects and seek answers to questions to prevent previous mistakes. It is an internal process. I divorced several times in my life. After the last one, I spent ten years being celibate. I took care of Florencia instead of looking for another woman. This was very much a stage 18 of my life, a very internal silent process of my life. A clearing of sort, for and of myself, for and of people around me. A deep reflection where I wanted to go and be as a person.

Another possibility for Stage 18 is coma. There are many examples of people who after coming out of a coma completely transform themselves and their lives and renew all over again. It is Stage 18 that allows that to happen.

CHAPTER 10

Homeopathic Analysis Phases

From all the cases I've seen, beside the fact that autism is clearly stage 12 in its M.O., I have noticed cases share another feature. Just like Stage 12, it is an analysis feature and ultimately only helps with choosing a remedy.

Phases in homeopathy are a new tool brough to us by Jan Scholten. There are 7 Phases comprising a system of evaluation of an individual's feelings of belonging to a group. From not being accepted in a group to feeling rejected from a group. My observations are that in cases of autism Phase 7 is overwhelmingly present.

When there is a phase 7 aspect to a case there is a feeling of being an outcast. This makes a lot of sense to me as individuals on the autism spectrum feel like they are out of the group, in fact it is the nature of autism to separate, this is partly what is so heart wrenching about the condition. Each Phase has some overlap with Stages in themes but remain very different.

The feeling of exclusion is often present during pregnancy and is generally expressed by the mom within four different ways.

- The feeling of exclusion at work. Perhaps mom or dad got fired. Another way of feeling excluded at work is by being relegated to a more menial job.

- The feeling of exclusion with the family. The in-laws or the parents feel like this is not the right time to get pregnant due to family dynamics, religious or personal beliefs. The acceptance of the pregnancy is not outright.
- The feeling of exclusion from the husband. Perhaps the couple is experiencing difficulties and divorce is being contemplated. The announcement of the pregnancy is taken as an impediment to working things out or a forced way of staying. Either way the pregnancy is not readily accepted.
- The condition within the marriage forces a breakup or exclusion with one side of the family. This is seen when the couple must move away for work and the mom finds herself alone in a new place without her support system.

PHASE 1:
The desire is to belong to a group but there is much fear or trepidation of being accepted. The situation is felt as unstable. Since this is a new situation, there is no friendship, the feeling is that of feeling alone, feeling like a stranger.

PHASE 2:
One is accepted within a group, as if he has just signed up but the connection is fragile. In this situation one follows the rules of the group. The feeling is that of being unsure, do I belong? Not really or not yet. Generally during this phase one asks a lot of question. The feeling is of wanting to be helped to get up to par quickly like kids moving in college. So many questions and answers.

PHASE 3:
Now that the rules are known one must adapt, most commonly by being very pleasing. Giving too much, staying too much at the office, agreeing too much to avoid arguments to be accepted. The feeling is of being halfway in and halfway out. There are positives and as long as I behave well all is good.

PHASE 4:

The position within the group is assured. The feeling is that of being responsible and loyal. One feels needed and the center of attention within the group. This is a very stable position; the feeling is that of being valued.

PHASE 5:

The feeling of belonging is clear, but they feel they must do more. Phase 3 does to be accepted. With phase 5 there is an exaggerated attitude. "You can't live without me" type. There is a quality of too much. There might be pushy parents, must succeed type, always wanting more. The opposite is always true as well such as partying and having a good time. (Case one reflects phase 5 and 7 really clearly.)

PHASE 6:

Feels taken advantage of by the group. He has to give too much or compromise too much. He is not feeling appreciated, he feels he must do far more than should be required. To remain accepted, they argue their position. They feel they are just being tolerated or the group just tolerates them. Reversely, this is the situation when someone is being lazy and not pulling their weight for the group.

PHASE 7:

They feel expelled from the group. This is the unwanted child. Feelings expressed are very hard and cold. The feeling of rejection, of not belonging is very strong. "I cut the cord with these people", communication is very strained and there is much aggression.

As stated, some aspect of phase 7 is usual in cases of autism. The feeling does not need to be throughout the pregnancy, nor does it need to be strong or totally traumatic. It can be just a remark, but that remark is felt deeply, and the mom didn't forget. During consultation it might be come up simply as "I should mention that my mother-in-law told my husband; why is she getting pregnant now since she is still in college?" Mom in law might be perfectly kind but the question makes such an impression that it is not forgotten.

CHAPTER 11

Cases

All cases are heavily edited to reflect the most essential aspects but remain within the spoken language of the parent rather than written English. Keep in mind, that the initial consultation is three hours long.

I have a simple gradation system which is on a scale from 0 to 10 does the child have eye contact (E.C.), Spontaneous Interaction (S.I.) and Spontaneous Speech (S.S)? The number is chosen according to what I see on the videos parents send, what parents tell me, and the answers to the questions I send prior to consultation. I commonly write a comment next to the number. I use it as reference of where we started. Ultimately the purpose of this practice is to always pursue neuro-typicality when starting with kids under twelve years old.

Many parents may initially find the answers to the questions quite familiar. However, as you delve into the probing process, it may start to seem peculiar and seemingly unrelated to autism. Such a reaction is perfectly normal. As a homeopath who has had the opportunity to unravel many of the mysteries surrounding autism, I approach your child from a different and deep perspective than what you may be accustomed to. This allows me to explore neurotypicality in each case, which is a departure from the simplistic ideas of using remedies for "clearings".

The analysis I provide after the initial consultation and subsequent follow ups is not intended to be as technically exhaustive as what I might present at a homeopathic conference. Its purpose is to offer parents some insights into the consultation and not why I've chosen a particular remedy, but clearly notice Stage 12 and Phase 7 in the process. I understand that the selection of remedies will remain abstract and puzzling due to the complexity of both autism and homeopathy. It's important to note that this book isn't a self-help guide; rather, it delves deeply into autism and offers valuable insights for parents. If you have a keen interest in thoroughly studying homeopathy, I encourage you to do so, but I advise against using it as a treatment for your child.

It's important to emphasize that not all cases are "Surrogacy" cases, as I mentioned at the beginning of this book, I needed alternative methods of analysis and understanding to increase reversals. With this in mind the cases presented in this book illustrate the often misunderstood, undervalued yet profoundly meaningful homeopathic process from the initial stage of a case to achieving neurotypicality.

CASE 1 (5 yr. old)

MC:

ASD

E.C.: 9
S.I.: 4
S.S.: 2

The mom started speaking about her child as soon as we connected on Skype. She never provided me with the answers to the questionnaire sent before consultation. There was a pronounced intensity to her, and I am sure she felt the questions were useless, SHE had to present the situation.

She jumps right in.

"We were not planning on having a baby. I wanted to continue my studies. Medically my pregnancy was OK. Me and my husband didn't get along and I am emotionally broken down. One time he took me for an abortion".

"When I delivered, he was a normal baby. Doing fine until 18th month when my in-laws got into the matter and asked: "How come he is not talking?""

"We started OT and speech therapy. He has been with her for 3 years. He is saying a few things but not on par with other kids. His teacher says he is OK and friendly".

"My husband and I don't get along at all. He is not staying with me now".

"There is problem when my child is in a group. In conversation he is lost, he repeats the same things. He looks at me and repeats what I say. He seems eager to pray, 5 times day". He says, "Where fan?" and he points it out. He can answer some simple question "Are you hungry?" "Yes" but is completely blank most of the time. He is not age appropriately holding a conversation".

"He has a lot of repetitive behaviors. He is opening and closing doors and windows".

"He likes the sounds of church bells. He is headstrong and knows exactly what he wants. He does not do what other kids say or do. I must explain things to him. Once I do that it is a lot easier. We are all worried how age appropriate he is. When we sing "Happy Birthday" he shouts. He does not like it".

"He sleeps very well, through the night. He is still not potty trained".

"There are those fears in him. At the beach, he wanted to go in the sea. Now he is in school, he has swimming, but he does not like it".

"He has his own favorite songs and cartoon. He is not media addicted child. He leaves the iPad away".

"He loves his bike and football. He enjoys those sports, but he does not play them or understand much about the game".

"He likes to go places and shows he likes surroundings".

"When the weather changes he has easily catches colds or cough. His fever shoots up to 101. Now is Monsoon weather, he is OK. He gets sick mostly in winter. In November he coughs constantly, it is bad. He is not able to get the phlegm out. It is a hollow cough".

TELL ME ABOUT "CONSTANTLY COUGHING", PLEASE

"It shows on his face that he has a bad cough. Throat hurting. He coughs more when he is exposed to the wind. I keep the fan off. The fan irritates him".

IRRITATES HIM?

"The fan wakes him up. He gets cranky".

HOW IS HIS DIGESTION?

"He does not have a history of GI tract issues. He goes to the bathroom immediately after eating".

TELL ME ABOUT YOUR PREGNANCY?

"I was very mentally disturbed and worried about my life. There was no way I was going to terminate my pregnancy. We had huge fights with much abusive language. I wanted to break the marriage. My in-laws were very supportive, and I stayed in it. My husband and I don't get along well at all. I don't understand what is wrong. There were long periods we didn't stay together. In the back of my mind, I think I am a very emotional person. I really loved him, but I stopped eating and seeing anyone. I was mentally tortured. Out of the blue, he sometimes would stop me from visiting my mother or my friends. I had issues with his friends. He did not come home; he was with them all the time. I would ask him to not do hanky panky things. All these things were building in me, and we would start fighting and quarreling. I felt emotionally broken. I was not stable, but I wanted my child. I got up and built courage, but I didn't want to go on".

DESCRIBE YOUR STRESS INSIDE

"How will I support my child? Will I have to raise him single handedly? I felt totally left out, alone in this world. He left me high and dry. Being so emotionally distraught, not getting any sleep or eating. Just crying".

"I too have a lot of anger in me. I cannot share with others. I have a lot of things inside me. Most of the time it is within me. Whatever fights were happening I was not saying anything to anyone".

"My husband does not support me, the in-laws are. This has really broken me down".

"The father comes from time to time. He does not believe he is on the spectrum".

TELL ME MORE ABOUT BEING "LEFT HIGH AND DRY"

"I am not supported at all by my husband. He is not contributing one penny. I don't feel loved by him. I have never felt love by him. I feel I am a burden on my in-laws. At times I feel like I have depression. I try to keep myself busy, I do feel the vacuum that my husband is not with me. At times, I wonder why I was faithful for him. He calls me "a bad wife and a bad mother". I am too young to be left alone".

WHAT DOES "BAD WIFE" MEAN?

"He thinks I disobey him. I have totally given up having a conversation with him. There are no answers".

HOW ARE YOU FEELING PHYSICALLY?

"I work out regularly, now. I walk and stretch a lot. I was very active and never showed signs of tiredness though I was very sleepy when I was pregnant. I was sleeping so much, my feet started to swell. The doctor made me lose weight because I was 70 kg. At night I felt a lot of acid reflux, I felt better with rose syrup in cold milk".

YOU SAID YOU FELT "LEFT ALONE", CAN YOU DESCRIBE THE FEELING?

"Before I got pregnant, I would discuss even the smallest matter with him. He was my best friend. I had faith he would make a good husband. Whatever I confessed to him, like I had fun with my friends, he got back at me as if I were his worst enemy. I started to keep things to my mind and heart. He would listen only but when I needed him, he was not there. He started to get involved with another woman and partied all the time. Then he started to keep me away from his friends and his personal life. I felt his friends were more important than his wife. I felt very broken down".

BROKEN DOWN?

"I felt broken down during pregnancy. He was involved with a girl then. I was made the bad one. I didn't have proof and that got me irritated. Even with his friends who were my friends too, he would make me feel as I were an outsider, so I stopped seeing everyone".

"I was shattered. What is the future? Any chance of improving? My life ended there. I didn't want to do anything; I gave up on everything".

TELL ME ABOUT YOUR CHILD, PLEASE.

His temperament is headstrong. He cannot take a "no". There was a time he could not even hear "no". I had to turn my answers around for him to not have him react. We can't fool him about what he wants".

"He likes to do a lot of things he is not supposed to. He told his grand-mother "I give you one tight slap" (echolalia phrase from a cartoon)".

"He is not an introvert. He likes to go out and explore things. He likes to attract other people's attention. He loves to go to birthday parties, lunch, diner in restaurant".

"He tracts with his eyes. He is very well focused and knows what is happening around him. He looks blank particularly when he is tired or when we speak to him. When we quarreled, he used to laugh, now he is very concerned. When the father is here, he does not look at me when I come in. He knows there is a problem, and I can read the expression on his face".

HOW DOES HE PLAY?

"He does not like to share toys with other kids, but he can stay with other kids around him.

Every evening there are about 10 kids in the courtyard, but he does not play with them. He is on the side".

REMEDY
DYAKIA HENDERSONIANA 30C

Other possible remedies: VERATRUM VIRIDE 30C
ENTODON CONCINNUS 30C

ANALYSIS:
I choose to present this case because of the obvious, Phase 7 feature: Feeling excluded. Of course, not all cases are so obvious. Also, Subphase 5 of the father partying all the time is clear. The presentation of her child is

rosier, less factual than it truly is. Speech is virtually nonexistent. I don't want to give false hope, this case progressed very quickly, at the same time quick reversal is one extraordinary features of autism that should not be ignored either.

I am sure many would comment that somehow her stressful state during pregnancy justifies the diagnosis, but it is not so. Nothing during pregnancy justifies autism. We must be very careful of judgment and beliefs by extension that don't offer anything but prejudice and pain. What is experienced during pregnancy IS the child as described in the previous "surrogacy" chapter.

In terms of remedies, there are many remedies with "forsaken feelings". Camphora is one of them, but the forsaken feeling is that of floating in a very cold, dark place alone. Lost into oblivion. This is not what she is communicating.

One could think of Veratrum viride however that remedy would have affirmed herself with very strange, self-inflicted behaviors to increase the drama rather than diminish it.

This remedy was chosen for the partying, over the top behavior displayed by the father as well as the quality of the mother DURING PREGNANCY, the main feature being, my relationship is not working out. She also presented quite frantically, went straight into consultation without turning in the questionnaire ahead of time. Of course, it is a Stage 12 remedy as the M.O. was, I will be forsaken if I lose control of this relationship.

FOLLOW UP I (2 months)
"He would never answer. Now, he answers, I asked him "What did you do in school today?" "The teacher asked me to draw or write ABC's"

"Did you do it and finish?"

"Yes, I finished"

"What did you eat?'

"I had sandwich, I ate banana, I had some water".

"He told his father: "The movie was good, but I got scared in the dark.""

"His grandmother said, "You are my baby". He told her, "Oh no, I am my mother's baby".

"He has been expressing himself in words. At times, there is still a little bit of gibberish".

HOW IS HIS TEMPERAMENT NOW?

"When things are explained to him then he is OK. For example, I can explain that it is dark outside so we can't go out for a drive. We can reason with him now".

"The other day he came up to me and said "mom, can I have ice cream?" He is taking instructions from me".

HOW ABOUT HIS INTERACTION WITH OTHER KIDS?

"He plays with other kids; he talks, interact and shares toys with other kids. Reciprocation is happening. He used to play on his own. There is group play with more participation on his part".

"He is addressing other kids by their name. That was not there. He remembers all his classmates. He tells me this or that kid had a birthday today. He never did that before. Pretend play is good. He plays different games, the other day he was playing doctor with another kid. Earlier he could not even play with blocks. Last week I had to buy him another set because he plays with them all the time".

"He is much better with his bike. He is better physically. His health is much better now. He is not coughing. More awareness of his body and the surroundings. He also does not stim. Tracking with corner of eyes is much improved. Opening and closing door is gone. He also transformed it as in pretending as if it is an elevator door".

DOES HE TURN BLANK AS OFTEN AS BEFORE?

"Much less blank and appropriate answers".

IS THE FAMILY WORRIED ABOUT BEING AGE-APPROPRIATE AS BEFORE?

"There is improvement towards being age appropriate. As far as speech is concerned, he is now 80% covered. Clarity of speech is still a problem as well as potty training has not happened yet".

REMEDY
DYAKIA HENDERSONIANA 30C

FOLLOW UP II (4 months)
"I can hold a conversation with him now. He can tell me exactly what he has done during the day in full sentences, he is using his brain now. Full multiple back and forth, he is very clear whereas that was not there before the remedy. Much less gibberish and a lot more clarity".

"One issue: He is not taking class order. "Everybody draws a flower". Everybody copies from the blackboard. Sometimes he does and other times he does not.

Second: He touches and leans on other children's shoulders".

"He is almost potty trained now.

He is very attached to his father; he gets upset when he misses him".

"He shouts much less. Still likes elevators. Not so excited about church bells".

"He is very social now. He has said he wants a birthday party and knows the kids he wants to have over. He is more social than before and participating. He was not participating before we started. Other kids also reciprocate".

HOW ABOUT BEING BLANK?

"I don't see him blank at all anymore. May be at the end of day when he is very tired, but we removed the afternoon nap so he goes to bed quickly too now".

"There is no stimming behavior except a little bit from the corner of his eyes. Not opening and closing doors. He does pretend to be coming in and out of elevator but that is different".

REMEDY
DYAKIA HENDERSONIANA 30C

Nine months after we started, he was diagnosed off the spectrum.

CASE 2 (2 yr.)

MC:

ASD

E.C.: 0 (He does not look at the camera when we take a picture. He'll look at the selfie afterward).

S.I.: 1 (He is the one chasing. He can get really focused on a truck but does not play. If we take a puzzle piece, he grabs all of them. Basketball hoop he will get, but he'll focus on something for less than a minute).

S.S.: 0 From time to time he says "up" when going up the stairs.

1: What unusual behaviors, interests, obsessions, tastes, aversions, fears - does your child have?

He is a happy child when he is around me, his father and grandmother. He is nonverbal. If he learns a word, I may hear him say it once and not hear it again for weeks or months. He does not point for items he wants. He does not respond to his name. He is a very hyperactive boy. He climbs on the table. When excited or bored he runs back and forth in our living room and kitchen. He usually smiles while doing this, then runs to me, my husband or his grandmother and hug us. Sometimes he spins around in a circle. He seems not to like shoes and socks on his feet as he takes them off as soon as we get home, in the car and at his daycare. He sometimes walks on his toes. He started biting his shirt and randomly bites objects. I realized when we ruff house with him or tickle him, he has great eye contact, but when we try to play with a toy that he is engaged with he does not give us any eye contact and turns his back to us or takes the toy away from us if we try to play with it. He has no eye contact when we talk to him. He may place objects that he wants in our hands but does not give eye contact. He does not point for things that he wants, instead he just cries. Joshua likes to line toys and other objects up. He then packs them away and goes back to the toys when he's interested again and lines them back up.

He tends to be interested in different toys. He will play with a toy for a few minutes and move on to another toy, activity or watch tv. He likes physical activity such as when we ruff house with him or any play where he can run back and forth. This is when he is the most engaged with us using eye contact.

I've observed him being obsessed with pushing the button on our fan to turn it on and off. At around 15 months he began wanting to walk around with his bottle in his mouth using it as a pacifier. His shirt becomes soaking wet because he tends to drool. I thought this was odd since he didn't want his pacifier as a baby and started spitting it out of his mouth at 3 months. He tends to hum and sings a lot.

Joshua eats different foods but must taste it first. He eats rice and peas, mash potatoes, green peas, oatmeal, chips, bread, spaghetti, chicken, and fish etc.

2: What makes your child upset or stressed and how does she react when upset?

He doesn't like to comb his hair or brush his teeth. He usually cries or tries to run away. If he wants something like the tablet or a toy and he can't get it, he will throw himself on the floor and start hitting his face. He gets upset when he wants food, or a bottle and he can't express himself. He also gets upset if he wants something to comfort him to go to sleep. He cries if he doesn't get a bottle.

3: What makes her calm, what gives her joy, what is she drawn toward doing, having?

He's calm when he watches TV. He's happy when he ruffs house playing or gets tickled. He likes physical play with other kids. He likes to play and stay in the vicinity of myself or his father or he likes to sit next to us while he plays. He also likes to climb. If I leave the room he's playing in, he follows me to whatever room I go to. If he gets upset, I hug him and that calms him down.

4: What are the main physical complaints of the child, how would you describe them?

Sometimes he will cover his ears when he hears noise.

5. Try to see life through your child's eyes. How does she feel inside? Consider the details --both good and bad. As a parent, you have a deep connection to your child. Pierre needs the information that you alone, as a parent, have access to. He will not need to see your child during the session.

He is overall happy. He gets frustrated when he can't communicate his needs and wants.

6. Reflect on the time of your pregnancy. How did you feel during the pregnancy? What was different during your pregnancy than at other times of your life? Was there any unusual stress, problems, issues, concerns, fears?

I had 3 miscarriages within 18 months prior to conceiving him. After my third miscarriage I was referred to a Chinese Acupuncture doctor. I began acupuncture weekly appointments; she gave me a tea I had to drink twice a day. Within five months I was pregnant with him. I was 39 when I conceived him. When I started going to the doctor, I felt like they always referred to my age and reminded me of the different risks for women my age having children.

During the first trimester of my pregnancy, I had high anxiety. I didn't want anyone to know I was pregnant and only told two of my closest friends. I became more anxious as the doctor began doing genetic screening tests and the results came back as high risk. I was then referred to a genetic counselor who talked to us about amniocentesis. I then switched doctors to a female. I felt more comfortable with her since she had a low C-section rate. She had me take a different genetic screening test and the results came back clear for genetic abnormalities.

I always felt doctors and hospitals try to push C-sections on women especially older women, so this gave me anxiety in my third trimester. My due date was in the beginning of September and leading up to that date I had no feeling of him coming on that date, I had no contractions, and my stomach did not drop. My doctor wanted to induce me, but I chose to wait to see if he would come on his own without intervention. After being a week overdue, I went to a doula who gave me a massage to encourage labor. The night of September 10th my water broke. When I arrived at the hospital, I still was not feeling any contractions. My labor was then induced, and I was given Pitocin. His heart rate began to go up and down. I tried to stay calm, but I kept looking at his heart monitor. After hours of being in labor the nurse decided to take me off the Pitocin since it seems like he could not tolerate it. I was in labor for 26 hours.

7. Can you say with any degree of certainty did your child have adverse reactions to a vaccine? Please list the vaccinations in order of adverse reaction.

He had 2 vaccinations; I do not believe he had any adverse reactions. Hep B, Tetanus.

8. Describe in detail the digestion of your child. Particularly the stool. Does your child test positive for any organism in the stool?

He takes a probiotic every morning. We put the probiotic powder in his milk. He's been on a probiotic since he was an infant. He usually has 1 bowel movement after breakfast in the morning and a 2ⁿᵈ when he comes home from school. His stool is usually soft and light green or brown in color.

9. Please provide Pierre with a list of medications that both parents were on prior to and during the pregnancy.

I was on pre-natal vitamin, fish oil, vitamin D, activated vitamin B, biotin, probiotic. My husband did not take any medication.

TELL ME ABOUT THE DELIVERY, PLEASE.

"When he came out, there was meconium all over the place, he was all green".

"I never felt contraction until they induced the labor".

"They kept alluding to C-section. Pitocin or not he didn't want to leave the womb, he wanted to do it whenever he wanted to. He was comfortable. I talked to him "we are waiting for you to come out". He does things on his own time".

"He sat up high through most of the pregnancy. I was running around and exercising as if he were part of me. It was not a problem. He was doing what he had to do. At 36 weeks his head was still up and at 38 weeks he did it. He did it when he wanted to".

He has always been happy and hugging and giving his family love. I am doing what I want to do. His dad was playing. He wants to do by himself. He hands it to us and then goes about his business. I want to be in control because I am me. I am laid back and I want to do what I want to do. I see the world as being busy".

BUSY WORLD?

"Right now, I am comfortable. There is excitement. It is warm and cozy in here, I can hear, I am so comfortable where I am at though. The world will be there when I get there".

AT THAT MOMENT WHAT DO YOU EXPERIENCE?

When I came out, I felt shocked. I got pushed out, wait, I was not ready. The world feels empty. Where do I fit in".

"I am feeling alone. I was comfortable having two in one. Now I am alone".

WHAT DOES "TWO IN ONE" MEAN?

"Strength. Strength is comfort".

DID YOU HAVE ANY FOOD CRAVINGS?

"I ate a lot of watermelon".

"Smoked herring. Dry. The smell is strong. It is pungent. It takes over the room. The taste is so delectable with tomatoes and onion, I could eat that morning, noon, and night. I felt satisfied".

DID YOU FEEL HUNGRY DURING THE PREGNANCY?

"Not much. For the most part I felt like I was getting prepared for the delivery. I strongly wanted to go all natural. Me, a bed, and delivery. It was

THE LANGUAGE OF AUTISM

upsetting when I could not do that. He had already pooped. I was upset. I had a plan, and it didn't go that way".

WHAT ELSE CAN YOU SAY REGARDING YOUR SON?

"He likes to be in the room with us. He won't stay in a room by himself. He makes sure he is next to us. Right by my hip or foot, he also loves my husband's chest".

"When I was pregnant, I was very distrustful about anyone talking about intervention. I thought they were after something else than my wellbeing".

REMEDY
BERYLLIUM NITRICUM 30C
Analysis: I gave this remedy because there are few issues during pregnancy. She is only looking forward the delivery. Phase 7 is there in term of firing one doctor and getting another. At delivery, the baby does not come, there is a significant delay already, but she is not concerned, even during the birth. "Hi, we're waiting for you". Delay is beryllium part. The nitricum part is the desire for watermelon, a fruit that is part of a botanical family that either grow very large or grow so fast some explode and herring, a very fatty, strong-tasting food is also an indication of nitricum.

FOLLOW UP I (One month)
"IT SEEMS AS IF WHATEVER WAS BLOCKING HIM HAS BEEN RELEASED".

"He has more eye contact. He does not have as much sensory issues. He is not spinning or toe walking as much. There is not as much "rrrrrrrr" when excited".

"He initiates play. He can bring something to me whereas he would just stay with whatever he had before. He never initiated help before. Now, it is 50 to 70 % of the time. I can also prompt him to look. Before, he would never turn or respond to his name, he is turning 50% of the time. Other people in the family have noticed".

"He has said "cat" "dog" On certain words he has started to echo us. Look at the banana and he says, 'nana'. Only, in the past week he has started on this base of progress".

WHAT ABOUT EYE CONTACT?

"He understands he needs to give eye contact in certain situations. The speech therapist says she noticed a difference with eye contact and his play seems much more appropriate".

"He is in the kitchen; he pretends to have eggs in the pan, and he stirs. He plays with ice cream set and scoops the ice and tries to lick the ice cream. He has never done this before. Could not have done it before".

"He can play with Mr. potato head for at least 5 minutes. Leaves and come back to it".

IS HE HYPERACTIVE?

"He was bouncing off the walls before, much less hyper now and not spinning around".

"He is pointing at things. He also pointed at the cat and said "cat". When I point at things, he also points at what I am showing him".

"Lining things up is much better. He has not turned the fan on and off. Less hitting of his face. Much less tantrums"

"He is also riding his scooter".

REMEDY
BERYLLIUM NITRICUM 30C

FOLLOW UP II

"HE IS MUCH MORE AWARE. He is waving Bye consistently. He is engaging with us to play. He brings his toys and balls. He is playing games and able to do what we ask him. He is aware of his sister. He acknowledges and plays with her. He responds to his name most of the time."

"It all seems promising. He plays with a variety of toys appropriately. No longer lining things up. Not turning light on and off".

"Eye contact is so much better even with people he does not know. Yesterday, we went to a daycare, and he followed the lady around. She commented that he was imitating other kids".

IS HE HYPERACTIVE?

"He still a little hyper, he climbs but the running back and forth is much less. Spinning is also a lot better. More functional play rather than running or chasing".

"rrrrr" sounds are nearly gone. Now he is babbling to talk rather than just sounds".

"Tantrums, toe walking, hitting his face also nearly gone. Still some biting and chewing on thing are the same as before".

REMEDY
BERRYLIUM NITRICUM 30C (dose every 5 days)

Analysis: There are deep improvements across different key areas such as eye contact, social sphere, and behaviors. Healing is moving in the right direction; functional cognition is lagging though it is very early in treatment.

FOLLOW UP III - VI
"Right now, he has about 10 words. He is doing a lot of approximation. On the other side, he seems to be understanding more. Husband has noticed he is saying more words".

"He has been initiating play with his sister. He is playing appropriately with toys and robots. He is interacting more with other kids. Also sitting longer in his chair when they do sing along. Participating in social games".

"When he is running now there a purpose, he is not aimlessly running back and forth like before. Tantrums and hitting his face continue to be low. He is pointing to things now when he wants something or when he wants to show something".

"From time to time a little toe walking. Spinning in circle still happens from time to time".

FOLLOW UP X
"He has been accelerating. It has been a progression. It is ongoing. Imitating more. Communicating his wants "I want cookie". He responds to his name all the time".

"Biting and chewing is finished. Spinning, very rarely. Hyperactivity is also very rare. No more running up and down. Toe walking is finished. On rare occasion he hits his face".

"His appetite varies, it is not a big issue".

ARE EYE CONTACT – INTERACTION AND SPEECH DEVELOPING?

"YES. Now he seems to say word. He understands most words of commands far better. He gets them and he can say words of commands as well. They are saying he is doing much better".

"HE IS A LOT MORE AWARE OF HIS SISTER. Yesterday, she was fussing, he went to her and put his hand and rubbed her stomach".

"He counts with the TV. He is pointing at things. Tapping me and showing me".

"No issue with toe walking, hyper-activity, or eye contact at all.

"Parallel play with other kids which is appropriate for his age. He plays with his cars, puts the driver in the seat. He drives them on the floor. He has other toys he plays with; it all seems appropriate".

"Speech is coming along. He is repeating. When I ask him to say something he'll repeat. "He points and says "Cookie, cookie, cookie" and I tell him "It is pretzel", he'll say "OK, pretzel".

"When he wants a toy, he'll give it to me and say "help". Before he would just put it in our hands".

"Progress over the past month. He is expressing somewhat clearly. What is new is that he is understanding language. He is trying to talk WITH PURPOSE".

"HE UNDERSTANDS LANGUAGE MORE. He is clearer when he requests but it is still difficult for him to put two or more words together. He is repeating and initiating "dad" He can repeat a sentence when we ask him. He can say his colors. When he watches something on TV, he says some of what they say. He understands, the sounds have meaning, not just making sounds. He understands what we are saying, this is new".

"He is meaningful when he hugs or kisses. He sits down for circle time. He is very interactive, engaged and playing with other kids. With his sister he is more engaged too. He brings her a toy when she cries. He pushes other kids away to be with her".

"He is showing interest in doing what his father is doing. At home he is not playing by himself.

His activity is not disruptive, can't call it hyperactivity".

FOLLOW UP XIV
"He still needs prompting and a lot of gibberish. "Mommy close the door" he wants to say it but does not come out every time. They are telling me that in school he is talking and in daycare as well. He gets the point of the stories he listens to. He is saying words and then we can understand. He uses the words correctly".

REMEDY
CALCAREA CARBONICUM 30C
Analysis: I find that language should be improving faster, so I changed the remedy to Calcarea carbonicum, a very common remedy I actually rarely give.

FOLLOW UP XVI
"HE IS COMMUNICATING. Not full sentences, he is putting two words or more together".

"I know what he is talking about. He says a lot of single words. He follows directives well".

"He played well with older brother and other kids. He has good overall comprehension. He is better than a month or two ago. He communicates more with us".

REMEDY
CALCAREA CARBONICUM 30C

FOLLOW UP
"Speech, he is starting to talk. "We'll drive around the neighborhood", he says, "look, Christmas light". His Eval says "spontaneously one or two words" needs to be prompted for more complete sentences.

REMEDY
LITHIUM NITRICUM 30C
Analysis: I went back to the previous remedy that helped so much. I've learned over the years this is a better choice than automatically move on to another remedy.

FOLLOW UP XX
"HE IS VERY CURIOUS. Asking questions. What is this?" He'll repeat the word that I say. When he does not know he asks. He asks what and where questions. "Mommy, where is my tablet?" "My toy needs to charge". "Where is Clara?"

"I am seeing length of sentences increase".

He is potty trained now.

REMEDY
LITHIUM NITRICUM 30C

LAST FOLLOW UP TO DATE
"He is not grinding teeth, not spinning or biting".

"We don't always understand what he says when we ask him to repeat, but he is speaking in sentences most of the time".

"He was re-evaluated off the spectrum. They say he only has a speech impediment".

REMEDY
LITHIUM NITRICUM 30C
Analysis: On videos, he is totally engaged with sister and others. He plays and speaks of Easter egg hunt.

Handwriting tells the whole story. Most letters look good.

Yes, speech will continue to improve but I won't be totally satisfied until he even drops "speech impediment" which I am certain he will.

"Sounds makes sense" that is key, and the handwriting is good. Total agreement with "off the spectrum" diagnosis.

CASE 3 (3yr. old)

M.C.:

ASD + Sensory disorder and speech delay.

E.C.: 0

S.I.: 0 (Never interacted with other kids)

S.S.: 1 (A word here and there if we prompt him)

1. What unusual behaviors, interests, obsessions, tastes, aversions, fears - does your child have?

He likes to throw things repeatedly ... but it has come down a bit, he is cranky when things don't go his way, no fears as such, aversions to experimenting with food textures.... very few kinds of food he likes to eat i.e.: rice pancake, porridge, biscuits, spicy food, rice, and mashed veggies, he is a vegetarian other than clarified butter (ghee) no milk products. He eats basically wheat free sugar free and predominantly vegan diet. He does not like social interactions with other kids and strangers and lacks eye contact but it's much better since his diagnosis because we are interacting a lot with him.

2. What makes your child upset or stressed and how does she react when upset?

He screams in high pitch voice when he is upset, and cries but then we can divert his attention and he stop crying... he likes to go out a lot so when he sees his father or mother leave, he gets upset and howls.

3. What makes her calm, what gives her joy, what is she drawn toward doing, having?
Outdoor activities like kids play area, going to park, roaming in the city in a car, roaming in malls... very peaceful when we go out... hardly cries.

4. What are the main physical complaints of the child, how would you describe them?
No physical complaint as such physically his body balance is good, no toe walking or stimming, no repetitive behavior, very active kid. He likes running around and explore nature.... doesn't talk though... but every day he is picking up new words through speech therapy and has echolalia .... in all he has said around 15 new words.

5. Try to see life through your child's eyes. How does she feel inside? Consider the details --both good and bad. As a parent, you have a deep connection to your child. Pierre needs the information that you alone, as a parent, have access to. He will not need to see your child during the session.
I feel he feels frustrated cause he is unable to express how he feels or express what he wants... he is very loving child, loves be around his parents, like structure in routine, loves going to school and watching things go by.

6. Reflect on the time of your pregnancy. How did you feel during the pregnancy? What was different during your pregnancy than at other times of your life? Was there any unusual stress, problems, issues, concerns, fears?
Due to the nausea, I was very week and most of time in bed couldn't walk around or go out. In the last three months, I was much better, I was quite stressed out because of my older son ... because he was not quiet getting adjusted at school.... but overall, it was not bad.

7. Can you say with any degree of certainty did your child have adverse reactions to a vaccine? Please list the vaccinations in order of adverse reaction.
Honestly, I feel like it all started with MMR injection given to him, around Feb 2020, for almost 1.5 YEARS I AVOIDED THIS POISON

BEING INJECTED TO HIM... TILL THEN HE DIDNT HAVE DEVELOPMENTAL delays as such... he walked on time, had social interaction, made eye contact, and had around 50 words in vocab, very active child... I didn't want to give him this injection, pediatrician forced me... it's not compulsory in India, and it's given in the 9th month but since he was 2.4 years and no sign of autism, I agreed... I felt my older one had developmental delays after his first shot... I know after this no vaccination other than hepatitis will come anywhere close to my children. I can't get over this guilt especially after avoiding it for 1.5 years.

8. Describe in detail the digestion of your child. Particularly the stool. Does your child test positive for any organism in the stool?
We haven't done any test as such... I feel his digestion is ok cause he eats healthy and mashed food mainly but now we are introducing new food. I can see there is constipation now. He prefers to have diapers that it takes time to pass motion. Now he can be in a corner and do it.

9. Please provide Pierre with a list of medications that both parents were on prior to and during the pregnancy.
I took aspirin and medication for thyroid (hypo) throughout pregnancy... I avoided medication altogether otherwise.

TELL ME WHAT HAPPENED, PLEASE.

"His brother had speech delay and was stimming, but he had eye contact and he pulled through. He had meltdowns. Now, I see a lot of similarity. Until April he would come and read with me".

"Post April he stopped going to school because of Corona. He could recognize mouth, nose, and recognize dad, or nanny. He would read a card and be able to recognize a lot of words and repeat them. Before April he was a happy child. In the last 4 to 5 months, he seems to be lost."

"He started walking at 15 months".

"He was potty trained at 1.2 yr., then 4 to 5 months ago he started to prefer doing it in his diaper and started to have meltdown doing on the potty. Now, when he is upset, he likes to sit in the car".

HOW IS HIS SLEEP?

"He wakes up around 12AM. He screams in the middle of the night; we turn the TV on and watch TV with him. The meltdowns started around 2 yr. old and now they are becoming more evident in the last few months. The sleep pattern was fine until 1.6 yr. old. He could sleep well. We'd change his diaper and then go to sleep".

"Now he wakes up around 2AM or 3AM during the night for a few days. His eyes are wide open and staring around, looking around and then goes back to sleep. At times, he wakes up at 5 AM".

"Yesterday he cried a lot. He was very cranky and didn't want to be touched. He wants his father to go away. Does not want him around in the same bed. He touches my stomach and navel; he recognizes it so with other people he knows and cries".

"There are days when he looks so frightened with his eyes tightly shut. He screams high pitch it is scary. When we sleep in the guestroom he does not sleep well. He is not afraid of the dark".

"In the morning, I wake him up and he goes to ABA therapy".

HOW WAS HIS FIRST YEAR?

"He had viral pneumonia when he was 10 days old, Antibiotics (ABX) and hospital for 10 days.

After ABX he had a severe yeast infection. We gave anti-fungal medication".

"Then he caught an infection from his brother. Cold and throat infection".

"He had foot and mouth disease at 1.1 yr. old from brother as well. That was the last time he was really sick for a year".

"When he went to school, he started to have cold and cough, we gave him a lot of Paracetamol.

Since lock down he has not fallen sick at all".

TELL ME MORE ABOUT YOUR PREGNANCY. DID YOU HAVE ANY DREAMS?

"My memory is quite weak in general and for my dreams and nightmares as well.

Something happens to my loved one or child. I am generally scared of death. Weird dreams".

"It is about being trapped, very scary and I try to wake myself up. Fear of dying". I also had, dream of going back to school or during my workdays. I was quite sleepy. I could only escape my nausea through sleep. I'd be in my night wear all day".

"Though I wanted a baby I felt I should have waited a few more months. Then I was fine with it. I was having a hard time adjusting to my older son. I had very bad nausea. I was unable to eat food. I was very worried getting enough nutrition. I was by myself, I felt if my husband could spend time with me I'd be happier. I wished he'd be more present given my condition".

"I didn't know what time of day it was. I was waiting for the pregnancy to end. I used to wonder that when the baby comes, I can't be in this position. I wondered if I was slipping into psych disorder. I felt like I was floating in the air, I could go and jump off the balcony. I never spoke about it with my mother".

TELL ME MORE ABOUT THE FEELING OF FLOATING IN THE AIR.

"I would lift my body up and fly through the hallway and then jump off the balcony. Some other force would pick me up and pushed me off the balcony. It felt good, it was a very nice feeling".

EXPLAIN GOOD, NICE, WITHOUT USING THE WORDS "GOOD AND NICE".

"I was able to release myself. It was a very repetitive thought. I was in a very monotonous thought. Feeling lighter and external energy lifting my body. I am more peaceful, and I speed through the passage. I can feel the speed and power of the push. It is very smooth and then the body is thrown off. It is not about my body colliding with the ground. It is a very abstract way of being. Then the energy is scattered, splattered but not in a violent way. No blood, no violence. It dissipates. I don't have body and bones, just a form of my body. A spiritual form of it. I never felt the thought was wrong".

SCATERRED?

"JUST SPLASHED but not on the ground. My ears were kind of blocked. I could not hear what I was saying. My body weight is lighter. I can feel it in my chest and heart. It is pushing out and contracting. Then it goes out, the energy disperses, and physical form ceases to exist, there is loss of time. It is not violent. It is more happiness. The energy floats. When I am going through the passage there are jerks and then it goes".

"During this pregnancy I hated needle pricks. I never feared pain so much. I didn't want to be pricked or anything to come inside me. I didn't want to experience pain".

TELL MORE ABOUT LOSS OF TIME.

"My mother stayed with me for a few months. She would tell me to wake up and freshen up. I just wanted to be free. I used to feel a lot of heat. My body was very sensitive to heat. During this pregnancy I could wear one layer of garment and feel hot. That continued post pregnancy for a few months. Even during the winter, I felt hot".

"During this pregnancy I could eat Indian food. I used to crave spicy foods like Chilies. I had specific craving for crabs. Spicy crab curry and rice".

"I cried a lot when I went out. At home I felt protected in that room. I felt comfortable in there. I even felt detached from my older son. It was more like an obligation. During the night I wondered if I would love my son more than the older one. I also thought I was having a daughter. I wanted a daughter. I always wondered if this baby was unwelcomed. I used to have tongue swelling when eating crab but not during pregnancy".

"I had crippling pain in the legs. As if something chewing on it. I even fell down. I was unable to walk. I had to be supported. I was fascinated by the pain. My leg would lose the feeling of pain. I could not feel my leg. I knew I had a leg, like paralysis but could not walk. From knee down I didn't feel my leg. I walked and fell. Shooting pain. Like a nail biting through the flesh. I was fascinated by the numbness, not the pain".

"It is like my son when he throws something. There is a kind of inquisitiveness. The numbness after the clinching I wanted to experience everything about it. See it. Wait for it, floating happened in my thought this happened in real time. I felt I was experiencing the weightlessness in my leg".

"Like the energy, expand and contract, the same thing as floating in the air. The numbness was shutting everything around me. The noise. The weightlessness of my leg felt good. The beginning of an addiction, I was liking it as if the body didn't exist. It never happened with any other feeling or injection this was a different entity all by itself".

WEIGHTLESSNESS IN THE LEG

"It is like LETTING THE BODY do what it naturally does. When my son throws these objects that is the kin-ness of my fascination with this feeling. I feel it now. Through sound he is experiencing something similar".

EXPERIENCE THROUGH SOUND

"He feels the sound. He likes it. the sound makes him feel this way. He wants to listen to it. It gives him some kind of pleasure. The pleasure is like the feeling I had. I can feel it now in my heart of contraction and expansion but not the splattering, but my son feels that. He gets that kin-ness. I didn't want anyone to come in my room and bother me. I didn't want to be disturbed. I enjoyed the fact that my husband was not around. I didn't even like my son coming in and talk to me. I liked being alone and not doing things. I had this fixation of reading the same thing, repeatedly, repeatedly, over and over again".

"I was reading a book about JFK assassination. I got a lot of books about conspiracy. It was a weird fixation. This was so weird. It was a representation of truth. I was so fascinated by truth. I ordered a lot of books about it. Read a lot of articles. I was unable to move on from that subject".

SLEEP PARALYSIS?

"My body is unable to move. I wanted to wake myself up, feet stomping, not ghost, I am brave, I cannot hurt me. The feeling of numbness is there again".

GO INSIDE NUMBNESS

"I am trapped. I can see everything around me but can't feel anything. I don't know if I can get out of it. I wiggle my toes, I can hear. Like being trapped in the body. The movement is not happening. Eyes are opened. Certain senses are opened, others are closed. I don't feel the touch for example. The balance is not there. I can experience the imbalance".

DESCRIBE THE EXPERIENCE OF IMBALANCE

"Being there yet not being there. The body is there yet it is as if I am not there. There is no balance. If it is not reality, what is it? It is very abstract again. I am on the bridge. It is a different form of existence. This is the bridge. It is where the body does not exist in this world. The crossing over of the bridge is the experience. The mind and soul are aware but not the body. Soul is trapped and unable to use the body. The lightness is there. It is not heaviness; it is existing but there is no feeling as such. It is the middle part. It is being there".

NO FEELING AS SUCH?

"Only what I can see. I can't feel the air and sounds. Alternate image. I only feel shadows, it is like a different dimension. I can hear and see it. Two images superimposed. I can hear the noise but what I see is super imposed. What I see does not match what I see. At times see shadow figure, I can see objects at times, but I don't know what is real. I can hear something fall but it is not there. I feel two worlds are being super imposed and I don't know which world I belong to. At times I don't know about dreams and the world. I try to figure out which world is real. I feel trapped because I can't feel the real word. The self is there but unable to move this way or that way, just the opening and closing, the release. It is very real".

REMEDY
ANHALONIUM 1M
Analysis: She call the pain "a different kind of entity". She is actually speaking about her son in utero. Cases don't get much clearer than this. She describes her experience during pregnancy, opening and closing and spontaneously connects it to her son. This is not a thought; this is after several hours of bringing her in tune with him through careful questions. This is not right brain creativity, this is a deep connection that runs her sensation in the legs, she sees it in his eyes and connects to it through his auditory sense. This is so exceptional to have several senses experiencing the same in two different people.

FOLLOW UP I

"He responds a lot more. His eye contact is up to 90%. He is quite clear when he points his finger now. He didn't' have that before, just a general hand gesture".

"Communication has improved a lot too. When he wants something, he asks for it with single words. He can repeat 3 words sentences".

"He still does not respond much to his name".

"He enjoys playing with his brother. He is playing catch. He watches his brother and follows him and imitates him. He is playful, he used to throw toys and wait for some sounds, now he plays much more appropriately with toys. 99% does not throw toys around".

"At his therapy center he is playing with other kids. He is also greeting other kids. He is learning to have people around him. He is not as aloof as before. He comes to look for us. He makes us part of his life now; he no longer sits by himself. He realizes when someone is missing. He is very aware of human presence and says other people's names. He seems to enjoy therapy and enjoys the learning process".

"Much less meltdown. He is repeating a lot of words. Does not scream much especially since the last week. There is a drastic change from what we discussed last time".

"He can say shapes, vegetables, and foods. His IQ is better than expected".

"Even the constipation cleared out and he is more regulated and every day he can pass motion. When he was taking a bath, he got out of it and sat on the commode. No need for diaper. He is not as gassy as he used to be".

"I can tell him what we are going to do, and he'll come with me rather than lead him to the activity we need to do".

"His sleep is also much better. Occasionally, he wakes up. Frightened and eyes shut during sleep is gone. He likes to sleep on my stomach with his hand in my belly button. When he wakes up, he takes my arm and says, "get up". He used to stare before going to sleep and that is also not there".

"He likes to be held, he likes a lot of hugging and cuddling. He seems very aware of our emotions. He wants us to be comfortable".

"He likes to go on a drive, but he does not ask people who don't drive. Ritualistic behaviors are going away. He would pick my shoes and I could not wear others. Those types of things are not a problem anymore."

"Physically his hair texture was really coarse, and he was very thin, he looks a lot healthier".

DOSED EVERY 3 DAYS FOR 10 DAYS AND THEN STOPPED.

REMEDY
ANHALONIUM 30C

FOLLOW UP II
"He has over 100 words now and can express himself. A week ago, there was a lot of echolalia. Yesterday we were walking, and he said, "I want to run". He saw a pillow and he said "sleep"". He loses his words from time to time when he is excited".

"He was so lost in his own world; he had 3 words. Now he wants company and most of the time stays with us".

"His sensory issues are gone. Removing his shoes etc. he does not do anymore. He does not have an issue with textures".

"Constipation but is much better. No more gas, he goes every other day. Once he did potty three times in one day. After that it started to regulate daily".

"He has not had any meltdown at all".

"I get scared when I give him the drops. After 3 days he suddenly talks a lot of words and then diminishes".

"He had severe lip cracks, but now it is gone. He used to have a lot of nose bleeds, but they have also stopped. He interacts with his brother a lot". He was generally a weak child."

REMEDY
ANHALONIUM 30C
Analysis: What I like about the progression of this case is that not only the language is picking up, but he is also associating. He sees a pillow and he says, "Sleep". These free associations are what I want to see during follow up.

FOLLOW UP III
"There is no dryness on his lips.

He is sleeping well, not staring at the ceiling for an hour is not there. There is no sleep disturbance either".

"Definitely the big improvement in language continues. He was never aware of me in the house. Now he looks for me and runs for me. He understands language in one situation and transfer to another situation. He can comment what he sees on TV".

"He can tell us when he wants to use the washroom. The bad smell of his poo is much better than it was. His motion is good. When he wakes up in the morning, he wants the diaper off and goes to potty on his own".

"He enjoys going out a lot. He likes to play with the keyboard. He plays with a child in his class".

"When he is in the car, he is always talking. A lot of commenting what he sees. Though there is a little bit of struggle to fully understand. He still repeats".

"Since last consultation giving the remedy more often. There is no dip in his development now.

He does not laugh unless there is a funny situation. He can emotionally relate to appropriate situation. He can have a good sense of kidding as well."

"He is not avoiding humans anymore. He was totally unaware. We are no longer objects. He knows everyone's name. He can comment which grandparent's house he wants to go to. He had no idea of grandparents before. Took him to grandparents for a few days. He like to play in the sand or water".

"He still has slight awkwardness in his body movement".

REMEDY
ANHALONIUM 30C

FOLLOW UP V
"Scored A.T. were 80 and now down to 22. His language has improved. He speaks with three words sentences in two languages. The language is not robotic at all. This month we have seen a huge improvement. He likes to sing rhymes".

Constipation is completely gone. Not wearing diapers. He used to have smelly gas. All of that has gone completely, his gut seems to have cleared out completely".

"Socially he is great. Just about neurotypical socially. He always wants his brother to be around.

His personality is really coming out and he can pretend to be playing with his toys. He can add his lines when he is singing. He is very Huggy, and very sensitive. If we tell him "No" then he still cries".

"He is gagging on food. He prefers mash food. Occasionally, he vomits.

He stims on the corner of his eyes. The whole family got together, and he was very good with the other kids".

REMEDY
ANHALONIUM 30C From time to time the dosing is more frequent.

FOLLOW UP VI
He is completely comfortable with full sentences. "I am drinking water" "I like water" "I am going to play". He is improving so fast, soon, in terms of learning he is on par with his peers".

With close dosing he is more responsive. When I started close dosing the sentence forming was very clear. It was a very clear jump".

"His aid is definitely in control of him but with us it is very difficult". He does not have any meltdowns at all". He is enrolled in a regular school".

"Before we came to you the doctor said there was no hope.

REMEDY
ANHALONIUM 30C

FOLLOW UP VIII
"I have been sip dosing once a week".

"Expressive is good. His sensory issues have dropped down drastically. Used to do eye glancing, now completely gone. He can use the stairs properly".

"Comprehension is good. He understands and answers all the questions we ask him. He is almost on par with kids of his age".

REMEDY
ANHALONIUM 30C

FOLLOW UP XI
"Speech has exploded, this month he lost the autism diagnosis. He is completely off the spectrum from two different doctors". "Very connected and lovable. He wants to meet new kids and acknowledges people. He wants to speak on the phone. He understands everything. These doctors told me he would never speak".

Once a day he is doing potty. Once the bowel movement got completely better his speech improved a lot. One day he did two poops that were really stinky, very badly and then OK. This was in March (Now September), rotten fruit smell, sweetish, I can still remember it. Like a jackfruit... BTW: he seems obsessed with jackfruit. He gets very scared of touching it. Wherever we go and speaks about it. He is afraid prickly texture".

"At times when he smells strong foods, he feels like puking. He does not like strong smell. Any strong smell he finds repulsive".

REMEDY
COLCHICUM 30C
Analysis: It is interesting that now he has an issue with pricking like his mom had during pregnancy. The choking or puking on food along with a slight stall in improvement made me change the remedy.

FOLLOW UP XI
"Though he was doing well, he kept repeating, his language is much better with this remedy. He is using full sentences. He understands and using elaborate words. His therapist assessed him for speech and he easily passed. With speech the jump is really evident".

REMEDY
COLCHICUM 30C

FOLLOW UP XII
His speech continues to improve, and he is doing well in school. He is grasping concepts very well at school".

"His ritualistic behaviors have gone away. His repetitions are gone as well".

FOLLOW UP XIII
"With Anhalonium there were autism qualities left but with this he is totally neurotypical. When the house is dark, he says he is afraid instead of walking through the house as if it were the same day or night".

"He is doing so well. He speaks two languages. His speech has improved and doing well in school. He is grasping concepts well at school".

"He does not fight nor any aggressive behaviors. He is understanding. He can report what he has done during the day. He can narrate a situation. I don't hear him make mistakes. He gets the concept of everything".

"Ritualistic behaviors are gone. He plays with other kids. No problems at all".

REMEDY
COLCHICUM 30C
Analysis: I look for total reversal. I have never told a parent their child needs a "clearing" of any kind. It sounds good to parents, as if one can magically clear something. I firmly think this is an excuse for not knowing what to do. While we can be happy with some improvements, I believe that my uncompromising attitude, and willingness to be fully dissatisfied with myself, even when some improvements warranted at least a smile, pushed me into the direction of successfully reversing autism. I have stayed away from ever saying to a parent that when a child is not doing well "It is detox, it is a good", Never! Because it is not true.

CASE 4 (4 yr. old)

M.C:

ASD

E.C.: 3 (Very shy, he goes between my legs when there are new people)

S.I.: 0 (No interaction at all).

S.S.: 2 (Repeats a few words and babbles. Doctors have told me; he will never speak)

1. What unusual behaviors, interests, obsessions, tastes, aversions, fears - does your child have?

He is obsessed with mickey mouse and dinosaurs he wants them all when we go to the stores. He also has a fear of dogs, he wants to be carried when we go to new places. For example, if we go to the zoo, he wants us to carry him the whole time, he refuses to walk. Also, he wants to be barefoot, not all the time he can handle shoes for school but when we take him to the park, he wants shoes off. He lines up his toys to play. When he gets mad, he cries, and flaps his hands really fast.

2. What makes your child upset or stressed and how does she react when upset?

He does not take "no" as an answer, he gets so mad, he hits mom and dad, he can get aggressive and it's really hard to calm him down. His tantrums occur when he does not get what he wants.

3. What makes her calm, what gives her joy, what is she drawn toward doing, having?

We calm him down by singing and rubbing his back. I also try to show him so many things until we guess what he wanted. What makes him happy is being outside in the yard, play with cellphone, watch TV. He also loves to line up his dinosaurs' toys.

4. What are the main physical complaints of the child, how would you describe them?
He has low muscle tone; he can't grab a pencil properly to write. It's been a problem at school.

5. Try to see life through your child's eyes. How does she feel inside? Consider the details --both good and bad. As a parent, you have a deep connection to your child. Pierre needs the information that you alone, as a parent, have access to. He will not need to see your child during the session.
The good thing about him is that he has a good memory. He remembers places, people, he can give sweet hugs and kisses to people he knows, he plays jumps and smiles most of the time. He sleeps through the night without waking up. He has some eyes contact he has made so much improvement on that. He is starting to repeat what he hears. The bad is that he does not understand our questions. He just repeats everything, he gets mad when we say no. When he tantrums he can get aggressive, he also does not play with other kids, he does not play properly with toys, he hits the TV when he gets excited. He has never had a haircut in a barber salon because he fears the machine, When I cut his hair, he cries.

6. Reflect on the time of your pregnancy. How did you feel during the pregnancy? What was different during your pregnancy than at other times of your life? Was there any unusual stress, problems, issues, concerns, fears?
My pregnancy was a surprise, my doctor had told me that I was going to have trouble getting pregnant because of my ovary cyst. We weren't expecting him. As soon as we found out we were having a baby I started having nausea and I vomited for about 4 months. I cried those 4 months very often because I was vomiting even when I drank water. In my 6th month of pregnancy, I was finally happy and calm; vomiting finally was gone. The 8th and 9th month of my pregnancy I became so scared for delivery I was not sleeping well I was so tired the last months of my pregnancy.

7. Can you say with any degree of certainty did your child have adverse reactions to a vaccine? Please list the vaccinations in order of adverse reaction.

I never say he had a reaction to vaccines other than a fever. I can remember the 2nd month and the 18th month vaccines those were the only ones that gave Julian a fever.

8. Describe in detail the digestion of your child. Particularly the stool. Does your child test positive for any organism in the stool?

He goes to the restroom every day; he never has a problem with stool or digestive issues.

9. Please provide Pierre with a list of medications that both parents were on prior to and during the pregnancy?

Dad has never been on any medication. mom only took Tylenol for pain.

When he was one year old, he didn't have eye contact. That got better when I removed dairy. He drank milk all day, nothing else. After two weeks he had better eye contact, he was more aware, and easier to please.

Milk was Similac and then milk. He was over feeding on breast milk as well. By six month he was a chunky, chunky baby. He gained a lot of weight.

With breast milk and Similac he had good eye contact.

IT SEEMS LIKE HE WAS CRYING FROM THE TIME HE WAS BORN, IS THAT CORRECT?

"He always had tantrums. He always cried a lot. He didn't let anybody carry or touch him except for me. He cried so much, waking up at 3AM until 7AM. At one year old he babbled".

"He crawled on time. He responded to his name when he was one year old".

"He rarely got sick, when he turned two, he started to have ear infections, throw up at night, and cough as well. When he threw up it was like jelly. It was a strong smell. The vomit was super-hot, strong like rubbing alcohol, acidic smell. I changed the brand of milk and it stopped. With Similac he was coughing too".

"At six months he was OK with other people but then at 8 months he started to be fussy again".

TELL ME ABOUT THE PREGNANCY, PLEASE.

"I got married in July, came back from the honeymoon with pain. I went to the doctor, and they found a cyst. I was told, I would have difficulties getting pregnant. So, it was really a shock that I got pregnant. After two months, I was vomiting so much. I started feeling better around the fourth or fifth month".

DESCRIBE FEELING "SHOCK", PLEASE.

"It really dawned on me that I was pregnant, only after the third month. When I started to get better my husband wanted to be with his mother four days a week. I had a hard time with that. My belly grew, I was happy to be pregnant, but when I was with my mother-in-law, I was mad. I felt he didn't' want to be with me, and that he was not comfortable with me. I felt lonely, but as soon as we were home, I was all perfect".

"I have a phobia of roaches. I saw one while I brushed my teeth. I screamed and cried a lot. I cannot see a roach even far away from me, I felt so hot, I could not even tell him it was a roach".

DESCRIBE FEELING MAD AT YOUR MOTHER-IN-LAW'S HOUSE?

"Disappointed and mad, I thought he wanted to be with me, he'd tell me, 'Let's go to my mom's'. What is he thinking? I didn't tell him I didn't want to go. Even now I never told him. "Let's go to my mom", it was so heartbreaking. I was crying in the shower from being mad. We stayed all day long until late in the evening. He didn't want to be with me, I thought he was not ready for married life. I felt I didn't love my husband as much. I am pregnant of him! I was so mad. It was all inside me. I didn't like my life at that moment. I felt lonely. I felt sad".

YOU FELT LONELY – SAD

"His mother came first. I wanted to get an ice cream, or a corn, he was not doing enough for the marriage, I was not pretty enough for him. I was growing big. We were watching movie without any conversation. Maybe I should study, I felt ugly at times. My nose got big too".

"Many fears came to me. My son won't have a dada or a family. I felt he would take my baby away. He also started to drink. At this moment, I think my son will want to drink when he is older. We were not working together enough. The biggest fear was divorcing him. I didn't want that to happen, and my baby deserves a dad".

AND YOU DIDN'T SAY ANYTHING AT ALL?

"I didn't say anything because I don't want to hurt him. We work now more as a team. I am grateful I never said anything, I thought, if I tell him the way I feel he may not want to be with me. I had a fear that he would say I love my mom more that you. I want him to be with me because I love him. When my son grows up, I also want him to come visits me when he gets married. I love him so much I don't want him to feel sad or guilty".

DID YOU HAVE ANY DREAMS

"No dreams while pregnant".

DID YOU HAVE ANY FOOD CRAVINGS DURING PREGNANCY?

"In the last three months of pregnancy I wanted pancakes, bread, and chocolate, mostly M &M. I craved sugar like never before in my life. Every morning I had to eat 3 pancakes with a lot of syrup".

TELL ME ABOUT YOUR SON, PLEASE

"He covers his ears when we go to Walmart, after 15 minutes he is OK. When we are with new people, he is OK after about 15 minutes too".

"He does not take "no" for an answer. He hits, he throws everything. He has so many therapies, and he still gets so mad, they are really a nightmare for me".

"I really want him to communicate, it is really sad. I want him to be able to communicate. He does not comprehend what I say at all".

DOES HE HAVE ANY FAVORITE FOODS? "He eats mostly anything, but vegetables. He can eat any kind of fruits all day long. He likes popcorn and peanuts. He has trouble holding a spoon or a pencil. Ever since he started school, he started to get fevers every month. He started getting sick yesterday. He has dry, white lips when he gets sick. He does not want to drink anything. Totally, thirstless".

Possible repertory rubric:

Complete 2020 Repertory > Face > Dryness > lips > thirst
✚ **With** (31) : *ang., *Ant-C, *BRY., *calad., *calc., *canth., *cast-eq., *cham., *chin., *clad-r., *cycl., *DIG., *geoc-c., *gins., *hep., *lachn., *Lyc., *meny., *merl., *Nux-M., *nux-v., *ozone, *phyll-a., *Puls., *rhus-t., *sac-l., *sulph., *term-a., *thal., *Verat., *zing.
(stomach; thirst)
Without, thirstless (16) : *ang., *arist-cl., *biti-a., *canth., *Caust., *cham., *chin., *cycl., *kalm., *kreos., *meny., *Nux-M., *nux-v., *Puls., *rhus-t., *thuj.

REMEDY
CARCINOSINUM 30C
NUX MOSCHATA 30C (second choice, but its grand feature is bloating which he does not have.)

Analysis: The mom in this case is so sweet, so kind, so emotional as well. Though I asked questions to fulfill the homeopathic process, she remained emotional, it was actually a very difficult intake. All remedies are confirmed correct or otherwise, through the results. In this case I did not know what to give. I gave this remedy thinking the enormous tantrums of the child were the other side of the same coin of the mom being so sweet and refrained, subdued, with romantic behavior DURING PREGNANCY fit this remedy quite well. This was guided by experience and instinct, at times homeopathy is also an art.

What this case demonstrates is that even if the remedy is not as accurate as in the other cases, for example in case 1; even missing the questionnaire makes sense and fits the case; well even when there is missing information, we can still achieve fantastic results.

FOLLOW UP I

"We have not seen much. He does not get upset as much as before. No tantrums for 5 days in a row but then he started again. Used to be twice a day".

"He repeated what other kids and moms said. "AJ don't' hit your sister" He was repeating clearly. He joined them for a short time. He was OK with other kids touching him".

"He is repeating things I say. Clearly repeating most of the time. He is expressing himself. "juice" "apple". He can also express certain feelings. "Leave me alone" "Play" "Music" He was not doing this before. Only communicated food wants".

"We went to his grandmother, he loves to be there, he said "mom, let's go home" Never said that before".

"He is also pooping a lot. He is trying some food, yogurt, and pancakes".

"He covers his ear because of the place he is in. He gets nervous when there are a lot of people. Still covers his ear =. Walmart or bathroom he does it.

REMEDY
CARCINOCINUM 30C

FOLLOW UP II – III

"The very first thing I want to tell you are the bad things. Throwing things or hitting me a lot. In school, we went to Valentine's Day party, and I saw him covering his ears most of the time and covers his face with his hands. One girl was telling him to come over and he was aggressive towards her".

"He no longer poops everywhere. "Mommy pipi. Mommy poopoo".

"He says more words. He uses English and Spanish. He plays somewhat appropriately. He also recognizes people; he calls them by their names. He calls us "Pappy" and "Mommy" he is not confused anymore".

"HE USED TO SCREAM ALL THE TIME. Now he is actually asking, he is laughing, he is having a good time".

"His program is to follow two steps directions; He can't really do that. I don't have conversation with him, it is sad. He understands pain. He says, "I have pain" Also getting feelings and emotion. When I tell him I am in pain he rubs and kisses me. I didn't know he could do any of this before".

"He does not like to go to school. He is not active there at all. It is actually difficult to get him to be active whereas at home he is very active. He gets annoyed with other kids".

DOSING EVERY TWO DAYS

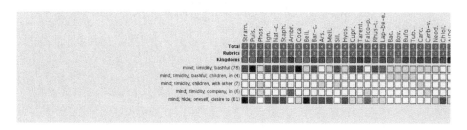

REMEDY
CONTINUE WITH CARCINOSINUM 30C.

FOLLOW UP IV - VII
"He has not improved since last month. He is hiding behind me and covering his ears.

"He knows words I didn't know he knew. Sometimes he speaks Spanish and sometimes English. He is pretty accurate in what he wants. But when I ask him "what are you doing?" He repeats the question. He is developing vocabulary but not responding to questions".

"The tantrums and his behaviors are through the roof. "He says "no" to everything. He wants to fight all the time with the toys too. He throws everything. Proper play with toys is challenging. He says give me the control "Mammy, give me for my toy" He knows the difference between Mc Do, Burger King, etc.".

"Attitude is still the same. Being contrary. Asking for one thing then another and then another. He is being very difficult. Even giving him a shower is hard. We had other children in the house, but he didn't want to share his toys. He plays for ten minutes at most with other children".

HOW DOES HE PLAY?

"To me ten minutes is a lot of improvement" He used to always be in my arms, and he didn't even look at the other kids. He could not even walk. He is also not afraid of dogs anymore. I have not seen him cover his ears. He says "hi" to other kids. He is having a lot of eye contact with other kids. He was always afraid of others. He brings dinosaurs to the other kids and wants to play".

"Giving the remedy every two days".

REMEDY
VERATRUM VIRIDE 30C

FOLLOW UP VIII
"His attitude is still bad, very bad manner. HE IS DEMANDING. "I want water! "Wait, Papy." "No, water". He throws a big tantrum. He fights a lot with the other kid. He only wants to be chased. He does not want to share his toys. He is like a dictator; he only gives orders and screams. At times he even refuses what he requests but he also makes mistakes in his requests, so he refuses because it is not what he wants".

"He is expressing quite well. He also gives a lot of eye contact and makes sure I am looking at him".

"He is eating all day long. He is pooping a lot. During the day he eats a lot of fruits. He loves lentils most of the time".

"He is understanding so much. His father told him he was going to work but he just wanted to go outside. He looked outside and saw the truck and told me; "Dad is still here, no work".

REMEDY
CARCINOSINUM 1M
Comment: The new remedy is not touching the behavior, that is a clear indication that the remedy is not accurate. At the same time, there is some cognitive development. There is a risk that changing the remedy will completely stall the slight improvement we are getting with Carcinosinum".

FOLLOW UP IX
"In the last 3 weeks he has done well. Last year was a battle to get him to school, I could not dress him, or put him in the car. He did not even go in the school. He was suffering. Now he is asking "Where are the teachers? Where is Ms. Ramirez? He is not using much language in school. Last year he was considered heavy autism. Now he is in leap but because he is not talking or tracing it is not possible. He is getting an aid for 4 hours a day. He has a good grasp so they are wondering why he can't trace.

He does not want hand over hand". They use a communication board in school, but he does not want to use it".

"People say they can understand him much more than before. He can answer a few questions, he is learning. But he still does not understand whether he is wearing a green shirt or red one".

"He does not mind being with other kids. He is very peaceful at school but not at home. Last Sunday he was hiding behind me and then after 30 minutes he played. He didn't hit the kid at all. "Go play with." "No, I don't want to".

"He is lining toys up. He names the toys and says what they are going to do". He says short sentences. "Turn off the light". "My tummy hurts". "Please give me the remote". "Pappy is that hot?". He is still repeating but using a lot of spontaneous sentences."

REMEDY
LYCOPODIUM 30C

FOLLOW UP XII
"He is playing with other kids. He is not hitting anymore. He is speaking in English".

"Not afraid of anything. A squirrel or a falling leaf he would run to me. He is not afraid at all. Also hated the swings, could not even look at them. Now he uses them on his tummy".

"He goes to bed by himself. Still some energy and jumping before bed. Much better before going to bed. He asks "mommy dormir".

"He is talking quite well. We don't have to guess anything".

"In school he refuses to do the work. He does not tell the teacher he needs to go to the bathroom". He shares and plays properly. He does not cry in speech therapy. It used to be a nightmare and now he is actually participating".

"At the grocery store, he can name everything and bags all the items. He was so impossible to be with this is so good. He is understanding everything. "I am a boy, I am xxx"

"He used to ask very rudely and had to be served quickly or he'd get very upset. Now he can wait and then he can come and say, "thank you". That means he is grateful.

He has scored low on reading test.

REMEDY
LYCOPODIUM 30C
Comment: He is not doing as well as he should be. He has progressed but not nearly as much as hoped. To a large extend we are still struggling with behavior, a clear sign that the remedy is NOT bull's eye.

FOLLOW UP XIII
"He is back and forth "I want to sleep, no I want to pee". He does it every day so many times, 50 times, I got upset".

"This month he didn't have a tantrum. Went to a family diner. There were kids and he played with them. He came to me when he needed to go to the bathroom. The kids were eating cereal and he came to me and asked me to take him".

"Played with toys and gave them back. He let everybody touch him. Give him hugs. Some people knew him for long ago and they could not believe how good he was".

"He communicated the whole time. Also requested to go to the toy room rather than always staying with us. He speaks in sentences. Mommy, I can't carry, it is heavy".

"His father says there is more difference with speech. He is saying more because of the TV. He is learning language through it. He repeats everything we say or tell him. He dreams and speaks during his dream".

"He does not jump up and down when he is excited. He is learning to use his bike and scooter".

He has not thrown a tantrum, but he still says, "shut up mommy". It hurts me so much when he says that.

REMEDY
LYCOPODIUM 30C
Comment: I want to be certain that when I change the remedy, it is a much better one than the current one. Lycopodium is not bad; it is just not great.

FOLLOW UP XVI
"He had a bad time after 4 days of not giving the remedy, so it should be repeated every 3 days to be sure he does not regress".

"Very good report from Psych, Pathologist" (speech therapy).

"He is answering questions. What was the book about? He could respond. "The book is about fruits". They say he is talking more.

"He also did not have any bathroom accident this month".

"Teacher, I need scissors. I can't do this, I need pencil". "Mom, I need to wash my hand. Mom, can I go to the bathroom. Mom, can I please eat..."

"The night is still a problem, it is my only struggle now, he refuses to sleep. He gets up and goes to bathroom, 30 – 40 times. He turns the light on and off. He pretends to go to bathroom".

(A possible rubric to use)

Complete 2015 Repertory > Sleep

Resisted, fight against (3) : bell., ferr., spig.

"He is trying new foods as well. He is also speaking with sign language. I never thought, what he is doing now was possible".

He can eat lentils. "No mommy, wait, it is hot".

"This is a boy, mom?" "Yes, pappy this is a boy". "Oh OK, Bye boy".

"Before he was in his corner and never noticed anything. He still gets stuck over minor things. We moved his car seat to my husband's truck, and he didn't want it. "Put it here".

"But I have to tell you, he had a huge tantrum. The police came "What is going on?" He cried for 5 hours in row. He had aggression. He is like this only with us, father, and mother; not with anyone else".

"His speech has improved. He is talking to me like never before. Other people have said, he is talking a lot more. In school they are very happy with him. He knows alphabet and knows verbs and subjects. He can conjugate verbs".

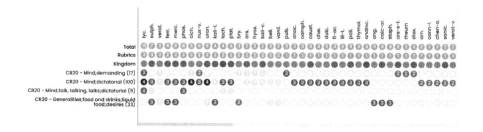

REMEDY
BERYLLLIUM NITRICUM 30C

FOLLOW UP XVII
"WITH THE NEW REMEDY HE HAS BEEN DOING AMAZING. He sleeps well and he is speaking more".

"Oh, booboo. Oh, it hurts?" he went to get a band-aid and asked me to put it on".

"The dog is not happy".

"No difficulty in bathtub at all. He is less dictatorial; he is at least saying what he wants. We went to the beach, and he had a good time. His aunt said he is not as shy and tolerates crowds. He seems to be getting what is right or wrong".

"At school he does not complains AT ALL. This is why he is not getting more services".

REMEDY
BERYLLLIUM NITRICUM 30C
Comment: This remedy is much better that the others. When in doubt, it is always best to wait. Giving a wrong remedy can have bad effects. Many people who claim to be homeopath give lots of remedies, often all at the same time. The potential for aggravation increases dramatically with such unprofessional behavior.

FOLLOW UP XX
"He is no longer fearful of animals".

"He still eats lentils, carrots, but trying yogurt, bread, chicken. I don't see any bad reactions".

"At school whenever we see the teachers, they tell us, he does not have any issue. The first day of school he didn't even cry. He is communicating and not using the emoji chart at all except to go to the bathroom. At school they say he is talking a lot. He says a lot of things, unprompted but short or in complete sentences. "Go outside. I want a blanket, mommy it's cold".

"Last year there were a lot of negatives. He only needs minor prompts. He can explain what he does in school. "I used the computer. I ate strawberries. I went to play at park".

"He is trying soup, spinach, lettuce. So open to new foods. "Mommy, it is time for bed". I am so happy with speech".

"When he gives orders, they are not like before. At this moment I am not scared to talk to him. He solves problems rather than getting upset".

"He has a couple of friends. Last year the school would send pictures, but he was always by himself, never in the group picture".

REMEDY
BERYLLIUM NITRICUM 30C

FOLLOW UP XXIII
"His disposition is better. The dictatorial ways are less. He used to throw things at me and tell me to "shut up", that is so much less".

"In school they say he is doing very well with other kids. He started reading. They went to the library, and he exchanged his books. He retains everything he sees and reads. "Mommy it is time for this book".

"He can actually wait now".

"Instead of chasing he can play with other kids. Playing doctor, kitchen etc. He can share his toys. He can also go upstairs with the other kids and play with them instead of staying close to me. He is enjoying kids now".

"He understands everything, He used to say "OK" to everything. He understands a lot more. He has a lot more variety in his answers".

"He still does not speak like a NT. He can answer every question but really short. He can explain but very short answers. He does not repeat the questions or repeats everything like before".

"He does not want to be bare feet anymore. He can wear different clothes. He goes to school in different clothes and does not mind wearing costume either for different events".

REMEDY
BERYLLIUM NITRICUM 30C

FOLLOW UP XXIV
"He has done brilliantly well with this remedy. He understands absolutely anything and everything. For 30 minutes he didn't move at all during homework".

"He can watch a complete movie at home without rewinding it. He never could go into a theater and now we go to the movies anytime we want. We could not do that".

"His dictatorial behavior is nearly gone".

"The school said they are giving homework now. He came home and he said "Mommy, folder trash". "No, Pappy, this is homework". Then he thought and was happy that the teacher was going to be happy the next day. So, he was thinking about the process".

"He gets consequences. If I don't clean up his toys, he gets that he didn't clean up".

"We have not seen a tantrum this month at all. Most of the time I have a happy kid".

REMEDY
BERYLLIUM NITRICUM 30C

FOLLOW UP XXV
"I WENT TO A BABY SHOWER: A few years ago, I decided I would never go to a party with him. This time, he sat in his chair, ate food like all other kids. He played with other kids. He followed the games he played with other kids. He didn't even know the other kids and he played without any issue".

"I took him to the bathroom, but he said "casa, baño" we went home, and he said, "baby shower, fun boys, so happy". I never thought this would be possible. Now he actually enjoys. He greeted everybody by name".

"Mommy, (I ate) potato chips (at the cafeteria)". He can say a lot spontaneously, but it is still broken."

"He went to a restaurant with his grandparents, he told me everything he ate. He also can handle being in a car without a car seat. He does not have a problem with long sleeves or hoodie".

"For the most part when something does not happen his way, he is OK now. He is also resolving his own needs. Used to be "Mommy clean up".

"They officially removed echolalia and non-verbal. Still on the spectrum".

"He does not say to "shut up" anymore. He is mainly OK with directives".

REMEDY
BERYLLIUM NITRICUM 30C

FOLLOW UP XXVI
"No Pappy, you can't do that". He gets sad. He is blowing me away with speech. "No mommy, I will call the police.' No mommy, I will go away"

Where are you going to go? "I will go outside". He is a lot of fun to be with."

"He is going with other people in the family without any problem at all".

REMEDY
BERYLLIUM NITRICUM 30C

FOLLOW UP XXVIII
"He is doing so well. This year he was able to participate at track and field with other kids. All good. His behavior is great".

"At this moment they teach him to read, he is on level B rather than F. "Dog jumping". You need to say, "The dog is jumping" "The cube is square" What did you do today?"

"He can answer all questions but not in sentence. He can also interact back and forth but mainly with two words sentences".

"He wants to learn in English not in Spanish, but he speaks in Spanish".

"He does not like to erase, he does not like to make a mistake, whenever he does something wrong, he gets upset".

Complete 2020 Repertory > Mind > Delusions, imaginations > wrong > he has done

People are therefore against her (1) : *lil-t.
(against him, people are)

(A possible rubric from the repertory that might fit this feeling).

"WHEN I DON'T GIVE THE REMEDY EVERY THREE DAYS THEN he takes much longer to fall asleep. He battles with his sleep when he does not have the remedy. He goes back to hyper-activity. Now he can sit on the couch and watch a full movie".

REMEDY
BERYLLIUM NITRICUM 30C
Comment: He is doing well on this remedy. The wise thing to do, granted experience helps, is to not give a remedy for this or that symptom, but rather stay with a central remedy that continues to improve the state as a whole. That is the only way to reach neurotypical. Keep in mind the possibility is for him to regress.

FOLLOW UP XXXIII
"I received another evaluation. The first time he was diagnosed with severe autism. On ADEC (Autism Diagnostic in Early Childhood) He started out at 176. Last year he was 120 and now 92. The cut off is 70. They cancelled Occupational Therapy".

"The evaluation from the hospital is better than from the school. There is a discrepancy that will probably disappear with time". Mother does not feel he is on the spectrum at all".

"Therapist says he does not need physical therapy. He can put a lace through or cut paper with a pair scissors. He could put a toothpick into a circle".

"He is not reading well yet, that is holding him on the diagnosis".

"He never tantrums in a store, have not seen it in a long time. He does not have any problems with crowds at all".

"He said he wanted a fish. We bought a fish, he named "Dolly".

"At school he still uses the chart in school only when he wants to go to the bathroom. At home he tells me but at school he is still using the picture chart. SINCE HE USES A CHART IN SCHOOL THAT IS HOW THE NUMBERS IS STILL ON THE SPECGRUM. They measure the weaknesses rather than the strengths".

"He plays properly with toys. He talks to the teddy bears. He also plays with other kids properly; I don't have to supervise him. He dresses himself. Sometimes his underwear is inside out, he says, "Don't worry mom, it's OK".

REMEDY
BERYLLIUM NITRICUM 30C

FOLLOW UP XXXVI

"I went to the doctor; he told me I have high Cholesterol. He saw I was distraught, so he asked me many times "Are you OK?" Mommy, go to the doctor" He is showing emotions. "Mommy, you need help? Do you want me to do the dishes" He helped me fold the laundry".

"He is requesting and does not get upset".

"He is dressing himself really well, he asks me if the shirt is right inside in. He was always putting right side out and when I told him he would get upset. Now we don't have that issue. He asks."

"He is drawing well, face with smile, eyes, hair, and ears. Coloring much less outside of the line. He can color with many colors.

"He needed to be prompted so much, for everything, he had no idea what to do".

REMEDY
AMMONIUM PICRICUM 30C

FOLLOW UP XXXVII
"Last month he had a field trip to animal park with turtles and crocodiles etc. I thought he was afraid of everything. He didn't have any problem; he even touched a turtle. He said everything he did. "Mommy I went to see the crocodile. I touched a turtle".

"OK, Pappy, let's go there again?"

"No, only with the teacher".

"He went with his grandmother to a park with duck and dogs. He took pictures of the animals. When he came back from his grandmother's he told me everything he did".

"He was at level "A" reading, he needs to be "F" and now he is level "E" and comprehending. On May 1st he said, "April is finish now it's May".

In school, he is very aware of the other kids and their problems. He tells me that other kids cover their ears, and he does not do it. He tells me that other kids have "tampers", and he does not. HE IS AWARE".

"There is nothing bad to say about his behavior anymore. He goes to bed without a problem, he is not jumping all over the place. He understands everything. When we go to the movie, he understands everything".

REMEDY
AMMONIUM PICRICUM 30C
Comment: This is one of my longest cases, three years! There are so many good things here. Essentially, he is very close to being diagnosed off the spectrum. It took time, several remedies but this is how life presents itself. Mom has been optimistic, true to her first consultation, she is present for the monthly follow ups, always, and it has paid off. Her child, who was supposed to never speak, is speaking! The doctors told her she should institutionalize her child, that child will now be part of society and live a perfectly, wonderful life. No finger will ever be pointing at him.

CASE 5 (5 yr.)

MS:

ASD

E.C.: 1 (Very rarely happens, only if we take his face in our hands)

S.I.: 2 (Parallel and "Hi" only)

S.S.: 1 (Just a few preferences, "I want" not conversational at all. Does not reply.)

1: What unusual behaviors, interests, obsessions, tastes, aversions, fears - does your child have?
Restricted eating behavior. Too much interest in electronic devices (iPhone, laptop). Closes his eyes and ears. Restricted eye contact. Does not want to sit or pay attention. Always keeps moving. I feel as if he is in pain if we make him sit for 30 minutes or more. He holds the lower part of tummy, but he never says or indicates he is in pain. He likes to eat sweets and ice cream, chicken nuggets. No vegetables.

He keeps on getting eczema on left leg. When we apply coconut oil, it goes away.

2: What makes your child upset or stressed and how does she react when upset?
Non-preferred activity.

3: What makes her calm, what gives her joy, what is she drawn toward doing, having?
If he cries, mom sits him in her lap, gives a hug and he is quiet.

4: What are the main physical complaints of the child, how would you describe them?
No physical complaints. He does not want to sit still. Less talk and social interaction. Poor eye contact. Does not pay any attention.

5: Try to see life through your child's eyes. How does she feel inside? Consider the details --both good and bad. As a parent, you have a deep connection to your child. Pierre needs the information that you

alone, as a parent, have access to. He will not need to see your child during the session.
He feels frustrated if he is not able to complete a given task. Suppose mommy asks him to close the door and the door gets stuck, he will start whining.

He is very much connected with us, and his teachers. He does not initiate social interaction with friends. He says 'Hi' to strangers without prompting. But after initial 'Hi', he doesn't know what to do next.

From his perspective. He is a smart boy and has good memory with poor attention span, who gets distracted easily.

6: Reflect on the time of your pregnancy. How did you feel during the pregnancy? What was different during your pregnancy than at other times of your life? Was there any unusual stress, problems, issues, concerns, fears?
I was desperate to get pregnant as we were late. After treatment for fallopian tube problem, I got pregnant, but then had a miscarriage after 2 months. I was very depressed. Three months later, I became pregnant again, but I was very stressed due to financial and immigration issues. I used to have craving for sugar. Diabetes was not detected; and delivery was forceps assisted.

It was a full-term delivery. He weighed 6 lbs. at birth. After birth he had a fungal infection, he was treated for it. Before going to daycare, he was a healthy boy. At 1.5 year of age, he started daycare and had several middle ear infections. He received 6 rounds of antibiotics and ultimately got ear tubes in October 2016. Initially, he was sick all the time, but I was told it was expected when kids go to daycare.

7: Can you say with any degree of certainty, did your child have adverse reactions to a vaccine? Please list the vaccinations in order of adverse reaction.
He had a bad response to MMR vaccine when he was 18 months old. Immediately, 3 to 4 days, after vaccination he had intense diarrhea and

eczema was so severe that he could not walk. Red spot all over, topical cream for treatment. The eczema was on his butt. No pictures. After that we saw changes in his behavior. He stopped responding to us.

Big strawberry red patches on butt cheeks and hips. Not liquid filled, just bumps. He seemed to be in pain. He cried a lot. It might have been burning to him. After 3 to 4 days, it was gone.

DIARRHEA: Very watery, transparent. I can still feel the smell. I remember thinking this is not right. The smell was very acidic and pungent. Very foul as if something is rotten. Within a week everything settled down.

He was holding his forehead with one hand. He was really not in a very good condition. The other hand holding his tummy very low.

No reaction to DPT, just fever.

After that when he was crawling, but not like normal. He would push himself/dragging himself forward with his forehead on the floor.

Then he started to talk less and became less responsive. By the time he turned two it was very obvious to us that there was something wrong with him. He was very hyperactive.

8. Describe in detail the digestion of your child. Particularly the stool. Does your child test positive for any organism in the stool?
He used to be constipated all the time. Even now. He is potty trained. We are giving him psyllium husk. That is helping him going every day.

He does not try new food. First bite is always tough. We have to bribe him. It is always a struggle. He was treated for yeast infection. Stool test was not performed.

9. Please provide Pierre with a list of medications that both parents were on prior to and during the pregnancy.
Mom had hypothyroidism since past 10 years. Earlier she was taking 25 mcg levothyroxine, at time of pregnancy it was increased to 75 mcg.

Father was taking SSRI (Sertraline) one year prior to planning pregnancy.

TALK TO ME ABOUT HIM BEING HYPERACTIVE

"From 18 months he has been hyperactive. Before then we never noticed it. He used to go around in circle for hours and hours. Then we bought a trampoline and that helped but even now he does not want to sit. He is still going from one room to another".

"When he sits still too long, he holds his tummy. He tightly holds his tummy on the lower part and rocks side to side. It seems like it is just anxiety when he has to sit. He cries when he does not want to do something. I don't want to go, don't do it. Virtual class is very difficult for him, he cries.

(Here is an example of a repertory rubric with abbreviated remedy names. I may or may not chose a remedy from it but at least, it is indicative.)

Complete 2020 Repertory › Abdomen
Holding, supporting abdomen amel. (20) : *adon., *boerh., *carb-an., *carb-v., *chin-ar., *coff., *coloc., *dros., *elaps, *fic-i., *hydrang., *kali-bi., *lil-t., *mang-acet., *Med., *morph-me, *phos., *ptel., *Rhus-T., *tab.

"He cries with tears and screaming and kicking. He tries to kick me, like "stay away mom". Crying is not for long, just a couple of minutes. If I promise his favorite show, he'll sit". He screams. "No". With online classes he has to sit there for a long time".

"He is very restless and looks here and there. He needs to hold on to something otherwise he has to run. He seems to be in pain. When he is restless it is a similar expression as when he is constipated. I always think he has to use the bathroom; it is the same expression. The first impression is tummy ache. It is obviously intense for sure".

DESCRIBE TO ME HOW IT FEELS?

"It does not last long. He wants to hide, does not like us close to him. Always feel like it is gas pain".

DESCRIBE GAS PAIN, PLEASE

"He goes to his room and locks himself up or covers his head. This gets worse when he has to do activity. It is short lasting. After 30 seconds he is fine. Then the pain comes back, it is repetitive again and again".

"Cramping kind of pain. When he is in pain, he does not want us around him. "You stay away" and locks his door".

IS HE VERY THIRSTY?

"He drinks a lot of milk. Casein free milk. Almond milk. He drinks a lot of water as well. He drinks so much once I felt as if I was going to faint".

"He sleeps well. It is sound sleep through the night".

DID YOU HAVE ANY FOOD CRAVINGS DURING PREGNANCY

"I used to crave a lot of sugar all the time. I drank dozens of condensed milk cans. I felt very calm and relaxed. I could not control it, sugar used to lift my mood, I was very happy afterward. To me everything felt strange. Like eating or tasting metal. A strange smell, as if sulphur. Then it makes you thirsty which gets rid of the taste on the tongue. It is like oxidized metal taste. There is a little coldness in the tongue. The taste goes in and out with the breathing. It makes my mouth dry, also create nausea. The smell felt like curdled milk. I felt acidic, salty. I also thought there is a strange covering on my mouth as well. I felt stuck in a situation with a lot of questions but no answers".

TELL ME MORE ABOUT OXYDIZED METAL TASTE

"Like rusty. Bitter and tongue feels dry. The bitter taste in the mouth. I can taste that rusty iron taste".

TELL ME MORE ABOUT THE PREGNANCY

"It was very precious for me. Things didn't go as we planned and our future. After our first miscarriage we didn't tell our families until I was 6 months pregnant. I had nausea all the time. I felt, I should throw up and I'll feel good. It was a trapped feeling and restlessness was there for sure".

FEELING TRAPPED WITH RESTLESSNESS?

"I can't do anything. As if controlled by others, there is no way of solving it. I feel as if I am fainting. I used to lay down. I just wanted to lay down and feel good. I lay, wrap myself in blankets and wanted to be left alone. Just let me recover from this. Three to four times during pregnancy, this very same feeling happened".

WHAT CAN YOU TELL ME ABOUT HIS EAR INFECTIONS

"High fever, he cried all the time, he was lethargic, food intake decreased, he was always in her laps. The eyes were watery, and he did not want me to go. Then he was always lonely. We could see the sadness on his face, I was always at work and his skin was always very dry. He was sick all the time and always irritable".

DOES HE HAVE ANY FOOD DESIRES OR AVERSION?

"He likes bananas, sugar a lot. He does not initiates trying new things".

REMEDY
BRYONIA 1M Dry dosing.
Analysis: It is not uncommon for parents to remember a smell, a taste, something having to do with the senses, therefore providing a connection

to the subconscious, literally to me a connection to the Universe and instinctively know, there is something wrong here. This is very precisely where one should focus. Yet, in this case, there is a very strong feature similar in the mom during pregnancy and the child which is "Not wanting to be bothered, no movement; in his case not moving the abdomen, wanting to be left alone, irritated, and dry". The remedy we must start with is Bryonia which has all these features.

FOLLOW UP I

"He initiates conversation now. When he sees something or does something he initiates. "Look mama what she is doing, she is riding a bike". We just can't believe that speech would just come out like this".

"One day I changed the bedsheets. "Wow, this looks nice, I really like it" He never expressed his view or opinion. Also, he looked at my shirt and he said, "Do you like it mama, it feels good".

"He is also trying to talk to peers as well. He can't maintain this for sure, but they see an effort".

"It happens a couple of times a day when he says something like "I'd rather sleep than go to school".

"He wanted the phone, I told him "No" and he answered "No? say "of course".

"Instead of crying he is conveying what he feels. We have more hugs and out of the blue, "I love you mama" and hugs me tight. though it is short".

"He has not complained a single time about tummy ache. That is very obvious, not a single time. We used to see that so often. No complains about tummy ache".

"The teachers are not seeing any transition issues, he is not crying or showing any resistance in class. He still needs to be redirected".

YOU SAID TO ME, "I FEEL HE IS ALWAYS IN PAIN"

"We do not see that. He can sit in one place and do what needs to be done. He was not able to do that before".

ECZEMA ON THE LEFT LEG?

"Gone. No need for coconut oil".

HOW OFTEN ARE YOU DOSING?

"From week to week he has been getting better and better. I gave one dose and didn't repeat for two weeks, then a dose every three days. After the second dose he was much better but the first week he was not so calm. After the second week began to become more communicative etc. After the first week we didn't see any tummy complains".

DO YOU SEE LESS ENGAGEMENT AFTER THREE DAYS?

"No".

REMEDY
BRYONIA 30C

FOLLOW UP II
"We are dosing every three days".

"He is much calmer. He wants to initiate conversation, but it has not increased further. He is attending class. He pays attention. It is still difficult to make him do tasks".

"We are not seeing him in pain anymore since we started the remedy, he is not complaining about anything. He is not holding his abdomen. Even when he is constipated, he sits there, not in pain but still only goes 2 to 3 times a week. Used to 7 + days".

"When I initiate, how was your day? He replies. Eye contact is improved. We play the blinking game. Eye contact is good. He used to move his head side to side to avoid eye contact. He asks me to make faces and I tell him I don't know how, so he does it for me and then wants me to repeat it".

"He can trick us. He wanted to come in my room where I work. He slides his phone under the door and asks to open the door".

"Interaction in school. He does not hesitate. He can repeat what the teachers say, he was not doing that last month. "Daddy come downstairs and sit with us". He can convey a message. He also ran straight to his father when I needed help even though I didn't ask him".

"He can sit with me for prayer every evening for 30 minutes without messing anything up".

REMEDY
BRYONIA 30C – 1M

FOLLOW UP III
"He is making sentences. Imagination is improving. Interaction is improving. School performance is not improving. IQ is still testing low".

"He is more open at home. Eye contact with us is fine. He is interacting in school. With peer influence he eats other foods, but day to day he does not eat much".

HE IS NOT EATING?

"Mainly milk and cookies and ice cream. Not eating much food at all. He has gradually been decreasing for a month. He gets very angry if he does not get sweets".

"He is not constipated. He has been sleeping well. He still covers his ears".

REMEDY
KALI PHOSPHORICUM 30C (I)

NATRUM PHOSPHORICUM 30C (II)

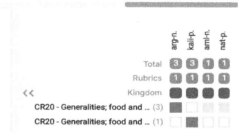

CR20 - Generalities; food and drinks; sweets; desires; irresistible (3) : Arg-n., aml-n., nat-p.
CR20 - Generalities; food and drinks; sweets; desires; only (1) : Kali-p.

FOLLOW UP V
"We are receiving notes from school saying he is very talkative and communicative. WE NEVER GOT GOOD NOTES FROM THE SCHOOL.

His aid says he can really control himself".

"Charlie, I like you very much, but I don't like when you hug me, so please don't". He is socializing as well. When he comes home, he tells us what he did. He describes everything. This kind of conversation is there. He replies in full sentences".

"When I read a book to him, he can relate to the story when we ask him questions. He was only able to use one word. Now he has difficulty with LONG SENTENCES".

"When he was looking for cookies in the kitchen, he would just whine about it. Now he says. "No, look in this cabinet, Ok, this one".

"He says "talk to me" if we don't answer his question. I can tell him, "Go tell your dad this or that" and he does it. He can take several multi steps directions".

"Sleep is really good, 10 hours without interruption. Not much problem

"He is not restless. When he reads a book, we can tell him "You can sit on the couch" and he does it. He is not restless while doing, same for eating and class. He used to run away".

"We still have problems with his eating. At school he can't eat anything. He smells the food first and then refuses to eat it".

"No issue at all with eye contact, he is starting to read my face and keeping the idea of expression. We are spending a lot of very good time together. We are not fighting, and he is not crying".

"No need to do hand over hand, he can write several sheets by himself now. Coloring as well".

REMEDY
KALI PHOSPHORICUM 30C

FOLLOW UP VI
"HE IS DOING AWESOME AND EVEN JOKING WITH HIS TEACHER. Story time is fun. He imagines in the book and makes up his own characters and action. He is talking on the phone with his grandfather. He told him that he hurt his thumb. "I got booboo in my finger" so he asked him 'how did you that?' 'I hurt myself on the treadmill.' 'Please put band-aid on it, OK grandpa'. He even started lying".

"He is helping me with the home cleaning. I rinse the plates and he puts them in the dishwasher. Same for the laundry. He was never that attentive before. He certainly would never have finished the tasks".

"He told me there is squirrel, she climbs the tree, and she has babies. "Mama what is she doing? What do you think? She is eating acorn?" We never discussed this kind of things".

"He started to write on his own. I needed hand over hand but now doing by himself. They are revising IEP all the time. The feedback is that we underestimated his capacities".

"He is attentive to what we tell him. Going to grocery store is so easy. Before he wanted to take everything and cried a lot. Now he waits to get in the car. At the doctor he followed all the directions. Everything, look here and there. Lift up your shirt. EVERYTHING he followed, never did this before".

"He can tell us the name of the other kids but at this moment we don't know because they follow COVID protocol. He is following yoga class and playing with stuffed animals even though he has had Donald duck for years now he talks to him and shows good inventive play".

"This is total magic for us. He used to take so many things. He even likes to take the remedy. He can remember Sanskrit and Hindu language".

REMEDY
KALI PHOSPHORICUM 30C
Analysis: Seeing such quick and deep results the parents were convinced he was no longer on the spectrum. They didn't consider the food issue as important given the lopsided improvements in cognition. On my end, a lot of details and questions remained unanswered. I am not fully happy. As far as they were concerned, he was fine and understandably decided to stop. To them, continuing to do follow up monthly to SEEMINGLY say the same thing and not change the remedy can seem like wasted time and money. Nine months later we restarted because speech was regressing, and overall improvement had stalled.

RESTART
"He is able to say things. "Give me a hug" "I want to go to the market"

He is interacting with other kids in school. He says "hi" he can get past that and "Let's go to basement" "Let's play". With us he is more communicative. "How was the class?" "It was good" "music". He can tell opposites. "Let's go to sleep upstairs" No let's go in the basement". He is somewhat awkward. He does not say anything we can't understand".

"He has constipation issue. I have to him a laxative. He won't go to bathroom for 4 – 5 days. "Massage my tummy" He bends a bit over when he needs to go, he seems to have the urge to go but does not. There is a bit of grunting. He is becoming a bit dominant when he does not like something. He is a bit lethargic when he is constipated. He has hardened poop. He becomes lazy when he has to go.

REMEDY
ASTACUS 30C

Complete 2020 Repertory > Generalities > Weariness > stool

Before (4) : *aloe, *kali-c., *nat-p., *rhus-t.
(stool; before)
During (15) : *Aloe, *Ars., *bor., *bufo, *canth., *coloc., *dulc., *hep., *kali-c., *lac
(stool; during)
+ **After** (20) : *Apoc., *bor., *bov., *calc., *carb-v., *graph., *ign., *lept., *lyc., *mag
(stool; after)
(weakness; stool; after)
Urging for (2) : *astac., *paraf.
(rectum; urging, desire)

FOLLOW UP X
"He is doing good in math. He is more involved with typical kids. He is transitioning well with other kids in a collaborative class. They make a team. He understands what is going on. They don' know he has autism, and they don't ask. He loves to go to school".

"As far as stool he is doing better. This past week, perhaps emotional growth and he gets emotional more than usual".

"He speaks in sentences. "I am Captain America" He is pretending to be such characters and taking the posture, that is new.

"Do you want to eat chicken nuggets "'No, I don't want to eat chicken." "Can you to market and buy chocolate?" "The market is closed" "can we go to market tomorrow?"

"Socially, he plays with his friends. "Can I go to Tom's house?" He can play with friends, but he is still missing some concept. He can kick a soccer ball a couple of times, and then loses interest. Still comprehending of concepts is not all there.

FOLLOW UP XIV

"He no longer needs speech therapy. They said he is able to reach all milestones and can reach them independently. He is speaking well. In school he is catching up, he can comprehend some books but may be not quite at his level".

"His stomach is fine now. He is not constipated. He is eating better than earlier"

FOLLOW UP XVI

"He is progressing especially math. He is doing math with advanced group. Writing is improving, he can sit and is very cooperative. His writing is improving day by day. Understanding is also improving. He used to write

A P P L E now he really writes apple as a word.

He didn't use to press much so difficult to read. He presses more and the letters are better formed. Still stick letters but before were very messy. He can write for a long time; he is not tired.

His teachers are very happy with him.

SPEECH

He tells me what is going on in school. He wanted to go to the bathroom, but he wanted to come home to do it. He told his friends, but they were laughing at him. "My friends were laughing at me". "Why were they laughing at you? "I told them I wanted to go to the bathroom but that I wanted to do at home."

"I told him to water the plants and he watered all the plants without me showing me how to do it. Then he came to me and asked me for $4 for doing it. Then he asked me if he could do more so he could make more money. He knew which plants he had watered and which he didn't, he differentiated with artificial plants as well that we have in the house, and he didn't make a mess".

Stomach is doing well. He is eating some of what we give him. For the most part he is good.

REMEDY
ASTACUS 30C
Analysis: When the mom said "now he writes "apple" as a word, I understood exactly what she meant. Handwriting is extremely important to me. One can almost tell if the child is still on the spectrum or not just by looking at the handwriting.

FOLLOW UP XX
"While we were in India, nobody said anything. Nobody suspected anything. Travel went really well, we went everywhere. He played well with all the kids. Super excited with his camel ride". For the first time he met his cousins, and he didn't have any problem. He paid great attention to what I was saying. He was very supportive and doing very nicely in crowded places. Covering his ears is not a problem at all, super cooperative. He did all his homework. Ate all kinds of food. Did not give us a hard time at all".

"Speech, conversing back and forth. He tells me everything. Speech is very spontaneous. At times I don't even remember he had a speech problem. He has more imaginary play too. He is playing a bit of basketball now. He understands the concept of putting the ball through the hoop. The kids didn't make any remarks".

"They think he won't need IEP anymore. At Kumon, he is doing math and English with a group of 5 kids. NO PROBLEM. His teacher says he does not need more help."

"There was something very satisfying to me. We were at a birthday party, and parents asked me: "Why he is on the spectrum since he is doing so well and so well behaved. You see, that is a sign that they over diagnose autism".

He used to have concentration problem and not at all anymore. It is straight forward for 45 minutes to an hour. It used to be such a problem.

In June he is starting piano.

He is getting ready by himself. Putting the clothes in the washer by himself.

REMEDY
ASTACUS 30C
Analysis: His handwriting is nearly off the spectrum. While he is not officially off it, it is only a matter of time within the next few months.

CHAPTER 12

A Complement to ABA Therapy

In the 25 years of laser-focused homeopathic practice on autism I have been privileged to witness and come across countless biomedical theories and therapy methods. A lot of fads have come and gone. To give you an idea, there was a time when parents were sending pictures of long jelly-like streaks in poop neatly exposed on paper towels to convince me they were "pulling" parasites, that they needed to be killed and that unless we got rid of them, autism could not improve. Not true! Every single time, I asked to get these things analyzed. On rare occasions, parents (of means) tested and every single time the results came back as negative for parasites. Parents insist but frankly, we know the features of parasites. We may not know which one it specifically is as so much has not been catalogued, but for sure any lab can tell if the matter is an actual parasite.

I do not dismiss the gut-brain axis at all. Before becoming a homeopath, I was fully invested in the supplemental biomed approach as my bio mentions. Nurturing bacterial gut flora, which rarely changes from birth, is far more complex than taking probiotics and regularly give an antibiotic for an ear infection or bronchitis or give an antifungal or anti-parasite medication as bacterial flora needs yeast to function.

Many parents take the road of supplements and medications to address "imbalances" and/or detoxify the bowel. The same idea holds true for chelation of heavy metals or heal the "leaky gut" syndrome. When I started 25 years ago, sixty rounds of chelation were necessary, now the average is well into one hundred. A conviction is real, but it does not make the parasites real nor do these ideas explain much as to why a two-year-old child is toxic with arsenic or heavy metals. The linear approach of removing heavy metals or parasites in a one-on-one fight seldom works because the complexity of the human body is grossly under-represented as a black and white matter to parents.

The cases in this book show us that homeopathy is difficult for people to grasp because the choice of a remedy is based upon the endless human nuances and remote from the very finite human thinking process of detox and supplements. Those nuances are absolutely key to restore health deeply rather than superficially. Human development is so extraordinarily diversified and complex, if we want to recover an individual from autism, it simply cannot be based on shallow one size fits all approach. Homeopathy does not point to a culprit such as heavy metals or yeast or parasites with a sleek color-coded printout of the supposed cause of autism. Rather restoration of spontaneous speech, interaction and eye contact rests upon a process that encompasses the totality of symptoms and individual as a whole and thereby restores the functioning of the natural stages of development caused by conceptual inability. When function is restored, the body can rid itself of parasites, heavy metals, etc. not the other way around. My interest is in the totality, as such my consultation goes back to pregnancy including the birth process, a moment that tells us how the baby was born, how and why interventions occur. We can glean a possible trauma from procedures, the mother recalls feelings, emotions, and experience. She can share the information she was told by the doctors. Nothing should be overlooked, as demonstrated in case 2, potentially all the information is within reach. It is only a matter of asking, understanding, and matching a remedy. Yes, indeed a remedy will match all of those, that is the beauty of homeopathy as well as its wonderment from people who don't know.

When it comes to speech therapy, the convention has a similar "black and white" or "head-on" problem. The approach is simple in thoughts. It basically involves sitting a child in front of a therapist. Get the kid's attention and try to imprint words or behaviors upon his brain. Often a less than convincing exercise.

While I am critical of these methods because they are incredibly simplistic, I fully understand parents doing everything possible "to get my child back". ABA is a method designed to get the child to say an actual "A" and upon completion of uttering the sound is given a reward, most often in the form of a piece of food. "I give you a cracker or a cheer" if you repeat after me, "apple" which is pictured on a card. "A – apple", "say A- apple" and the child is supposed to say "apple" and get a piece of cookie or a burst of excitement, "Good boy!!!" which today, often replaces the cookie. This was frowned upon years ago by parents fearing that their child was being treated like a pet, meanwhile, ABA became the main approved treatment for autism. If the child wants a glass of water, then the word is broken down to "wa" and "ter". Say "wa-ter" and I'll give you water. Fundamentally the approach is of the same kind as allopathic medicine namely to coax the body; in this case the mind and the will to pronounce words. The effectiveness of a medication is based on the similar principles of coaxing the body to do something it won't or cannot do. The goal is to coax the child to say a word. The child however has no purpose to say the words, he has no concept to say any word. Right now, that he is feeling thirsty he might blurt out "wa-ter" but that is it, most of the time he does not remember the word water a minute later.

This approach seems completely out of step once we understand that a child on the spectrum suffers from lack of conceptual ability. That alone precludes such approach. Then once we add to this fact that a child on the spectrum feels mentally overburdened to begin with, that coaxing or demanding more only aggravates the situation, then ABA truly seems out of step with reality. It is human nature to press, to coax, to force, to make something happen and to achieve results. We like to bend nature to our will, most of the time nature succumbs to our will rather than rise through it, so I fully understand the purpose behind ABA, but it can be made more effective.

The alternative

Speech therapy is not within my job description. Rather, my observations of alternatives to ABA led me to make an informal recommendation to "learn how to speak to a child on the spectrum" to parents inspired by Marci Melzer of Waves of Communications.

The first and foremost recommendation focuses on removing the stress from parents and children associated with speech delay or difficulties. Let's go back to the "water" example which can be applied to any of the multiplicity of other similar situations.

A five-year-old wants a glass of water but does not say the word, she only points. For years, she has been asked to say it but still cannot utter the word, she does not even try. After years of trying, it is time to change. Stop asking her to say "water". Imagine yourself being insisted upon for years to do something you are not able to do. For sure, you will get upset. The same principle applies here. Imagine being asked to repeat "D.d.d.d.-dog" over and over again. Without a doubt anyone will get super upset and even strike the therapist for being too much in his face. This happens all the time, and invariably the child gets blamed.

Instead of insisting to say water, which is not only boring but also frustrating for all parties, what I suggest is to describe water when the child takes the parent by the hand to the sink. "You want cold water from the fridge". "The water is going to feel cool going down to your stomach and it is going to give you the sensation of wetness in your mouth and tongue". "Once the water goes through your body you are going to pee". How much richer is that? It might become exciting for the kiddo to say something. Of course, this is extra, it is exemplary, but it acknowledges the child through sensations. Sensations don't use the brain; they bypass it. It is a lot less stressful. Even if the kiddo does not verbally speak, it is the start of a different relationship with the child. You are now building a "word savings account" for him. You are no longer in repetitious questions. You may feel he won't understand this long sentence. It does not matter so much because you are kindly educating your child. It is more than likely that your child will understand some of it. This is invariably what parents say. "He does not speak but I feel he understands everything." Exactly! And that is what we are going to capitalize upon. Gesture with your hands the water going down your throat and the cool feeling in the stomach. This is so much more alive than the static "water". You are associating sensation and speech over a word and a theme. This is an enormous difference, and you fulfill your one-on-one parenting.

This is what I call "speaking-through-the-senses". Let's take the color yellow, for example. It may take a long time to get the child to say "yellow" or even refer to what yellow means but yellow can very quickly be associated with banana, "The banana is yellow" but wait there is the smell of the banana, the shape of the banana, the taste of the banana. Suddenly there are several options to learn yellow.

In this context, yellow becomes experiential. Further learning can be connected to that, such as the stickiness of it. Suddenly, all the senses are used around the color 'yellow', some of it will have resonance with the child and some of it won't which is fine because when you notice resonance you are learning something about your child. "Yellow" may not get any traction, but the smell of the peel may. Let's see if the same holds true with something else then you know you can reach your child through smells.

Anything becomes a platform for speech. Most kids on the spectrum like to take car rides. Describe that a car has four tires, describe the smell of the seats, the feel of them is different from the metal of the body. Speak the experience, touch the tires, touch the hood with him. It is another way of exploring the world. The seats feel velvety with a different bounce than the hood.

Since a lot of children on the spectrum like to touch things all we are doing is using the expression of touch the child is attached to, to create a learning relationship and experience rather than say "don't touch". I believe ABA would be much more successful this way. Resonance is created by following the senses, as I wrote at the very beginning of this book, only resonance heals. This can be created anywhere, at any time. A cake is not only something that is eaten. Put it up to his ear and lightly squeeze it, the moisture in it creates a sound. Take a croissant apart and there is a sound.

The sounds transform into taste. All experiential, all make for richer interaction, more importantly everything becomes a potential. It may sound complicated and long but, all that is required upon hearing the sound of the cake is to say "yum", "it is moist". So, the experience can be long as with the example of the car or just an association of goodness through the word "yum".

A lot of children like to play with leaves and the same applies there too. The leaves are dry and crumple in the hands into confetti. Bringing this into his life builds great wealth he can draw upon later. Experience transcends conceptual inability.

As you implement this, you will learn more about your child's affinities as this becomes a two-way street. You can go where his affinities are and introduce more complexity. He may look the other way, but experience tells us that even when looking the other way, the children continue to absorb. Whatever you have time and energy for but do this consistently, over time his word and experiences savings account will be substantial as the homeopathic remedy restore conceptual ability, the words stored will come out.

I often hear "I didn't know he could say or understand..." By doing this, you guarantee that these moments become the norm and your joy will be mutual. It is quite baffling to me that a group of individuals who on average scores higher I.Q. are asked to say "water" when they are thirsty. Let's use their I.Q. as a tool rather than leaving it on the sideline.

As mentioned earlier speech therapy is not what I do but within all the years I have been in practice this is quite literally the only method I have deemed constructive. I have adapted the method to what I feel is more fundamental and effective. The end of the first consultation is generally taken by a short explanation of this method, and I urge parents to do it at every follow up, it is not easy. Since then, I have had countless examples of children qualifying their wants. One of the first one was a girl who said, "I want my pink shoes". The child added the word pink to her sentence. It may not sound like much but what is important is that she defined the shoes. She didn't pull anyone to the shoes or had a tantrum because the parents could not figure what she wanted. She defined her want. This is very early on, and she has gone on making much further progress. Finding a remedy that reverses conceptual inability, and unlocks developmental delays is possible, this method enhances those functions along quite well.

CHAPTER 13

A Red Flag System to Prevent Autism

With the particularly detailed and profoundly analytical intake required in homeopathy certain patterns mentioned in this book became recurrent in cases of autism. This is what inspired this burgeoning red flag system. From what I understand of autism, I do not believe a solution will be found in the lab. I believe a long-lasting reduction of autism can be achieved by connecting the dots from clinical, triage questions starting with the OB/GYN to the pediatrician.

This is a working theory. A lot more cases should be analyzed than I will ever be able to, to conclude whether all cases have the patterns introduced in this book. The red flag system I present should be understood as being cumulative. Being mindful of how single facts are often taken out of context of a whole, most often to advance a particular agenda, I want to stress that none of the red flags should or are responsible for autism, especially on their own. I do not have any proof that these red flags cause autism, so I do not make any claim, this is only based on my observations. If red flags lead to autism it is mainly through a cumulative effect. As such, I think it would be worth conducting studies that take a broader view of possible causative factors rather than narrow studies to single factors and let the evidence lead the results.

Red Flag During Pregnancy:

From the emotional plane:

1. An exclusionary moment either in the form of a short unfortunate sentence taken to heart from a family member or a sustained stress either from family or work. Another example is that of a mom who said she felt excluded as the only female engineer on a team of seventy men. This makes sense when we take the resonance with phase 7 (exclusion) into consideration. Autism clearly excludes, as is remarked in "He is in his bubble". A bubble is by nature exclusionary. The sentiment of being excluded, being an outsider is a central feature of autism. It therefore makes sense that the feeling of being rejected would be an issue on the external mirror, reflected on the inside. The pressures of abortion also come to mind as phase 7. It is not a factor by itself, there are plenty of kids on the spectrum with parents who were perfectly happy to have a child. In such a case that type of red flag is simply not present, but in the former the system should make a prominent note of it. Once again, it is not because a mom wants to get an abortion that the child will be on the spectrum, as I mentioned do not try to advance an agenda to create a controversy where there isn't one.
2. Failure to thrive in utero is a most important red flag. Underweight is a red flag. If from pregnancy one were to have an underweight baby together with a sustained rejection theme during pregnancy, that constitutes strong relevance not a certainty for the child to be on the spectrum. The system however should pay attention. We know that low birth weight has a five times higher chance of being on the spectrum than the general population of children of normal weight. My observations seem to be accurate.

There is a caveat to low birth weight. Are we thinking about this the wrong way? Is it the low birth weight or the medical interferences due to low weight and the further procedures that create autism? I understand turning the question on its head dramatically changes its content, but should we not investigate rather than take for granted that medical procedures are not contributing to the problem. I am not saying preemies or low birth weight babies should be left without care to prevent autism. What I think is that we can rethink those procedures to avoid catastrophic consequences. The challenge is that each procedure on this list does not cause autism, much like vaccines don't cause autism but only in very few cases; finding that has been supported by the vaccine court. Nothing is an absolute, from where I sit, it seems largely a succession of events lead to autism. What we unequivocally know is that the incidence of autism has gone up from 1 in every 2500 people in 1960 to 1 in every 38 people according to a South Korean study in 2011 conducted by Dr Young-Shin Kim. The CDC website page on January 9th, 2023, was "last reviewed on March 2, 2022" lists 1 in 44 in 2018, counts for 2020 and 2022 are not listed.

Red flags During delivery

The birth process is a hinge time of life. This is the time when parents, family and doctors focus on. A lot of thoughts, emotions and opinions are shared to prepare for that time. Many people make very concrete plans for it, which not uncommonly are very quickly abandoned for the safety of the baby.

In homeopathy, the birth process is broken down into eight distinct stages. Each stage relates to some specific remedies; therefore, I spend quite some time to understand not only whether there was a problem at any stage but also the emotion that each or one or none of generated.

Any birthing process has its imprint upon children and adults buried deep in forgotten memories and experiences. Given that autism is most often treated early in life the birthing process is still rather vividly on the mother's mind.

The following descriptions of the "birthing stages" as used in the homeopathic analysis of a child on the spectrum can be extremely useful to find a healing remedy. These "birthing stages" do not correspond to the medical definition of "Stages of Labor". Medically, the first stage of labor and its two phases correspond to the first three homeopathic birthing stages. The second stage of labor parallels the other 4 homeopathic birthing stages. Medical practice considers a third stage of labor which seems to be our phase 7 as it mainly with problems with expelling the placenta, or also heavy bleeding also related to placenta.

A history of issues during birthing stage 1 – 2 – 3 and then 7 in people with autism seem to be far more present than 4 - 5 and 6.

Birthing stage 1:
Premature birth, too late, past due date, the key here is that the birthing process does not start. It might seem odd to include premature birth in stage one, but it points to the acute, unprepared quality of stage which was described in Stage 1 M.O. Another possibility is the birth starts but then suddenly stops.

Birthing stage 2:
The position of the baby. All breech presentations relate to this birthing stage.

Birthing state 3:
The baby has not dropped.

The cervix does not open. At some point during delivery the cervix stops short of 10 centimeters. The birth can be delayed or even lead to emergency C-section.

During pregnancy, the opposite might apply as a stage 2 issue. The cervix does not close. Boron (which is the third element from the left on the second row of the table of elements represents that stage really well. is well known for acute hearing, perhaps due to a cervix not acting as an effective barrier to sound.

Fear of going down the stairs later in life relates to that stage or crying when lowered in the crib.

Birthing stage 4:
The contractions expel the baby but in stage 4 the contractions are weak. OR too strong, painful. These are the pain that make the mother cry or irritable during birth. The mother might begin to have great anxiety before a wave of contraction. In adult life this can translate in "anguish before menses" as the Materia Medica describes.

Birthing Stage 5:
This is the expulsion stage. The baby might get stuck in the birth canal. A shoulder has displaced the position. The birth stops. Quick decisions are taken. In adult life this can translate in having a fear of tunnels, tight places, or a desire for speed. As a child can be a very restless. Does not want his bedroom door closed.

Birthing stage 6
The breath! This is the blue baby stage for whatever reason.

Birthing stage 7:
This is the disconnection from the mother stage. There might be problem with umbilical cord, too short, or single umbilical artery which is the most common abnormality. There might be problem with the placenta. Placenta previa, for example or the placenta not detaching. Too early cord clamping could also be a problem. For example, lack of iron in the first months.

Abortion is also part of this birthing stage.

There seems to be an inordinate number of children on the spectrum who had either delayed birth, induced birth because of being at the end of the 40 weeks' gestation time. These observations are only from my practice and my cases. They only reflect what I see within my tiny vantage point.

3. A large head circumference at birth or soon thereafter seem to be a factor, dozens of research studies have shown a correlation, yet in 2020 a meta-analysis "Head circumference trends in autism

between 0 and 110 months" lead by Joel Crucitti suggested *"The present study cannot confirm HC to be greater in autistic than in TD participants between 0 and 100 months. Rather, we can conclude there exists a disproportionate frequency of extreme cases of HC in autistic than in TD males and females at varying age ranges. We conclude that future research should emphasize the variability of HC in autism, rather than comparing mean data."*

I am not sure how long and how many more babies heads we are going to measure, but for now, let's just take larger head circumference as a red flag and let's move on.

After birth, several flags can appear in quick successions. During consult I focus on the first six months, and then the next six months. Then I focus on the second year. The goal is not to determine whether the child has autism as all my patient are diagnosed. The goal is to search for symptomatology.

4. Is the baby latching on quickly? Never latched should be a red flag How long it takes for the baby to take the breast? If the baby is taking several days irrespective of the mother's production of milk, this is the next flag. The mother not producing enough milk is not as much of a problem as the child not being able to suckle.
5. If the baby can't suckle but easily takes the bottle, that is a flag.
6. If baby can't breastfeed and refuses the bottle that is a red flag.
7. The baby is colicky very quickly after birth. Red flag.
8. Does the baby have diarrhea often? Is the baby constipated? Both along with other flags should be monitored.
9. Is the baby sick or repeatedly sick in the first six months to a year such as frequent ear infection that are treated with antibiotics. Antibiotic use may play a big role in the development of autism.

Imagine this. A baby is born with failure to thrive. Does not breastfeed. Cannot be put to bed quietly, suffers from colic and develop ear infection.

When there is such an accumulation of red flags, this is when medicine should limit vaccination that seem to be the "push over" of interventions. With such a deterrent system, the mindful pediatrician could chart these flags and I suspect some cases of autism would be prevented.

Lexicon of New Terms

Autism Modus Operandi: The acting and reacting pattern of individual on the spectrum.

Autism reversal: When an individual on the spectrum gains so much contextual and specifically conceptual abilities there is no likelihood of being considered on the spectrum.

Birthing stages: Broken down into seven different steps, they define the process of delivery from the moment the water break (or not) and / or the beginning of contractions. These stages do not correspond to the medical stages of labor.

Conceptual inability: Absence of information processing. The essential reason of autism.

First witness: The mother who is pregnant is termed the first witness of the child since she is the one experiencing her own changes during pregnancy.

Functional speech therapy: The concept of speech therapy that inspired sensorial speech.

Interstitial space: The space where conceptual life and contextual situations are processed.

"One Heart, One Mind": My second book based on the "surrogacy case taking" method to treat an individual on the spectrum. The process is designed to bring voice to a child who cannot speak through a parent or significant other.

Parenting from behind: The method of parenting that takes into consideration the pattern of action and reaction of an individual, especially one operating from stage 12.

Phases: The seven phases of acceptance, belonging and rejection within a group or family.

Prodromal autism: The conditions starting during and after pregnancy defined by events and facts that may lead to autism if certain interventions are not avoided.

Red flags: A multi-faceted triage method that might prevent autism. Red

flags take into consideration prodromal autism conditions and after birth events to establish a sensible approach to the life of a baby to avoid pitfalls that may influence to development of autism.

Sensorial speech: A way of speaking through the five senses that connects inside the child with speech.

Stages: Each of the 18 stages reflects the way we act and react in life, in disease. Each stage has its characteristics well defined. Stage 12 is largely the stage of autism.

Surrogacy: Method of case taking that brings voice to the child who cannot speak, through a parent or someone close.

The language of autism: The symptomatology of an individual on the spectrum that at face value seems absurd but means something.

Three-legged stool: Colloquially defines autism as lack of spontaneous eye contact, lack of spontaneous interaction and lack of spontaneous speech.

- E.C.: Eye contact
- S.I.: Spontaneous interaction
- S.S.: Spontaneous speech

Appendix

Part two speaks about dosing the remedy using drop, sub-acute or acute dosing instructions. The following are the instructions everyone receives when we start.

They have been worked out over the years and in my view give the best basic instructions to dose a remedy. That said they are essentially guidelines and are not meant in any way to be rigid in the way a medication is commonly given.

It is my view that the dose must fit the case and that testing its plasticity is critical. I give the parents a lot of leeway in dosing according to what they "see and sense"; often they find a way that fits the child better than these three options. The same goes with the frequency of the dose. There too, I leave a lot of leeway, but old habits do die hard, and it is difficult for some people to not dose according to a specific day. "We dose every Sunday night." Whatever works taking a homeopathic remedy is not like taking a medication!

HOMEOPATHIC SERVICES, Inc.
Pierre Fontaine RSHom CCH
Classical Homeopathy Consultant
192 Lexington Ave (2nd Floor)
New York, NY 10016
212 334 7360
www.homeopathicservices.com

DROP DOSE Instructions

Here is the remedy and the instructions on how to administer it.

1. Place **one tablespoon** of water in a small glass (shot glass is perfect)
2. With a dry spoon take **one pellet** out and drop it in the water.
   It will take about 10 minutes to dilute. If it looks like it did not dilute then shake it up a little and it should blend nicely. Swirl the water a bit.
3. Give only **2 - 3 drops** from the dilution, **ONLY ONCE**. (Not once a day. Just ONCE.)
   Before going to bed with a neutral environment in the mouth. Neutral environment means it is preferable to not have any food, toothpaste, or juice 30 minutes prior to giving the drop.
   Please store the remedy (pellets) in a cool and dark place away from electronics.
4. **Email me 7 days later** with an overview at **Pierre@homeopathicservices.com**
   Be sure to observe your child closely and write a brief summary detailing his/her reactions 7 to 10 days from the day he/she began taking the remedy.
   Wishing you well,

HOMEOPATHIC SERVICES, Inc.
Pierre Fontaine RSHom CCH
Classical Homeopathy Consultant
192 Lexington Ave (2nd Floor)
New York, NY 10016
212 334 7360
www.homeopathicservices.com

SUB ACUTE Sip Dosing Instructions

Please hold on to these instructions until Pierre tells you to use

Please dose for ONE DAY only. After that ask Pierre on how to proceed.

1. Place **4 ounces** of room temperature spring water in a very small water bottle.
2. With a dry teaspoon take **one pellet** out and drop it in the water and let it dissolve. If it looks like it did not dilute then swirl it a little and it should blend nicely. **Shake the bottle vigorously 10 times.**
3. Give a **quarter teaspoon**. There is no need to refrigerate.
    Give one sip (one quarter teaspoon) 3 or 4 times per day. A quarter teaspoon in the morning, at noon, in the afternoon and at night before going to sleep. **Shake the bottle again before each quarter teaspoon. The dilution is good for one day.** Please store the pellets in a cool and dark place away from electronics.
4. Email me 5 days later with an overview at **pierre@homeopathic-services.com**
    Wishing you well.

HOMEOPATHIC SERVICES, Inc.
Pierre Fontaine RSHom CCH
Classical Homeopathy Consultant
192 Lexington Ave (2nd Floor)
New York, NY 10016
212 334 7360
www.homeopathicservices.com

<u>ACUTE</u> Sip Dosing Instructions

Please hold on to these instructions until Pierre tells you to use

1. Place **4 ounces** of room temperature spring water in a very small water bottle.
2. With a dry spoon take **one pellet** out and drop it in the water. Stir the water. If it looks like it did not dilute then shake it up a little and it should blend nicely. **Shake the bottle vigorously 10 times.**
3. Give **a sip once** (quarter teaspoon) every **30 minutes** or until symptoms improve. You can cover the glass with plastic wrap in between sips. **Shake the bottle again before each <u>quarter tea-spoon</u>.** You can do this anytime of day. Please make sure there is no food/juice in the mouth at the time you dose.

   The 4 ounces <u>does not</u> have to be finished. The dilution is good for a day and there is no need to refrigerate. Use a new pellet each day of sip dosing.

   Please store the remedy (pellets) in a cool and dark place away from electronics.
4. Email me 5 days later with an overview at **pierre@homeopathic-services.com**

   Be sure to observe your child closely and write a brief summary detailing his/her reactions 5 days from the day he/she began taking the remedy.

   Wishing you well.

About the author

P ierre Fontaine CCH RSHom has been a homeopathic consultant since 1994. He started seeing patient on the spectrum shortly after starting his practice and quickly developed a passion towards autism and the parents of children diagnosed on the spectrum.

Fontaine spent five years researching alternative health care, including herbal and vitamin therapy, detox methods, acupuncture, and ayurvedic medicine before finding his passion in homeopathy.

Fontaine has lectured on homeopathy at the Autism One national conference and at many colleges. He testified before the White House Commission on Alternative Medicine Policy. He is the author of several published articles most notably on MRSA. His first book titled tongue in cheek "Homeopathy, Sweet Homeopathy", opens the mystery of the professional practice to the general public following 38 cases of general illnesses. "One Heart, One Mind" the first book on the treatment of autism using homeopathy brings out the concept of surrogacy case taking, to bring voice to a child who cannot speak.

Websites where you can reach Pierre Fontaine

https://languageofautism.com
https://reversingautism.net

Thank you… to the World.

Made in United States
North Haven, CT
25 September 2024

57853163R00127